MANUAL OF

JOINT MANIPULATION

Prepared By
Byron E. Laycock, D.O.

Professor of Osteopathic Principles
& Practice

Des Moines Still College of Osteopathy
& Surgery
Des Moines 9, Iowa

1953

CONTENTS

Table of Contents (Cont.)

Table of Contents (Cont.)

Table of Contents (Cont.)

Page

CERVICAL AREA - PAGES 367-404

SHOULDER GIRDLE AND UPPER EXTREMITY - PAGES 404-437

PREFACE TO 1ST EDITION

This plagiarist has found no manual or text on manipulative techniques with what he feels is an adequate number of pictures to maintain continuity.

The desire is to accumulate enough such pictures in series of a sufficient number of techniques that this manual may facilitate the development of efficiency and accuracy in joint manipulation.

Realizing that every physician modifies orthodox techniques depending upon his height, age, weight, strength and alters those even when the same factors vary in patients, it is obvious that no single piece of technique will ever be adequate.

Still, the facet or joint surfaces and the area of the hypertonicity and joint restrictions will remain fairly constant.

The general principles of joint manipulation and the direction of the corrective forces will be the same, or should be, regardless of the great variation found necessary in practice.

A purpose of this manual is to attempt to demonstrate the principle of a technique and the direction of the corrective forces. The closer we can approach this physiological correction, the easier and less traumatic will be the essential correction of lesions.

Byron E. Laycock D. O.

FOOT AREA

CONSIDERATIONS OF PROPER FOOT GEAR

It is not platitudinous that the super structure and all its functions are conditioned by the first plane of support. Hence, uninteresting as they are, the shoes and feet of every biped are an even 100% more important to him than are they to a quadriped. Look down from several dozen feet height and watch people walk. Note - just **HOW** they walk, nothing else. When a person walks, he walks with every articulation in his body: arms, hands - and am sorry to say, often his tempero-mandibular articulation. This locomotion phenomenon has a greater effect upon the individual than it does upon you.

The shoes form the contact that keep the feet "fitting the limb", and preventing them from completely resembling the immediate contact, the very hard and very flat concrete.

Shoes have a definite mechanical function and they may be altered to influence favorably the super structure, statically and dynamically. In outline, shoes must fulfill the following requirements.

REQUIREMENTS OF A GOOD SHOE

1. Form a resilient, not hard, cushion between the foot and the walking surface.

2. Sufficiently large that it will not deflect the toes nor impinge the interosseous tissue, when **ALL** the weight is on one foot. Must be symmetrically fitted.

3. Be so constructed that it will distribute static weight bearing in the essential percentages. (See chart page)

4. Have a comparatively rigid outer weight bearing arch that will not permit the shoe to twist around its long axis.

5. Have a flexible inner spring arch that will permit normal weight bearing arch descent.

6. Have a heel height over the sole that will maintain a lumbar index of 1-1/2 inches.

7. Straight last shoe.

8. Provide adequate ventilation.

Outside of these considerations it matters little whether the shoe has an enclosed heel or ankle straps, whether the toe is in or cut out of the shoe, whether it is made of grass, leather, wood, or waterproof cardboard.

2

STATIC WEIGHT BEARING
IN GOOD FOOT MECHANICS

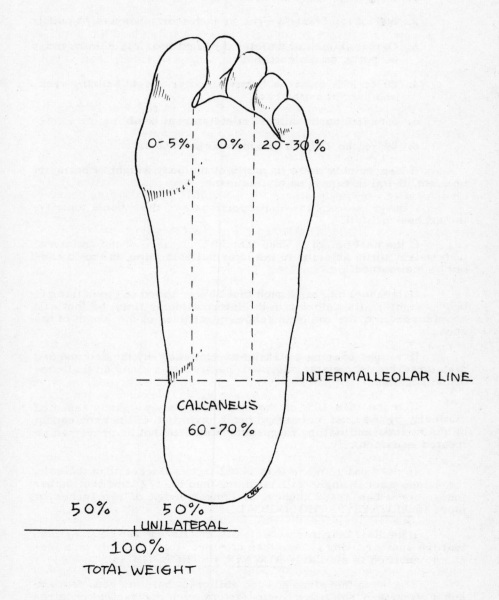

0-5% 0% 20-30%

INTERMALLEOLAR LINE

CALCANEUS
60-70%

50%   50%
UNILATERAL
100%
TOTAL WEIGHT

STATIC WEIGHT BEARING

The foot is poorly designed for prolonged static weight bearing. If it is to maintain good foot mechanics, a definite pattern of distribution of such static weight is essential.

1. Feet must be directed straight forward.

2. 50% of total body weight on each foot. (See weight shift)

3. Of that amount of unilateral weight bearing, 60-70% must be borne on the calcaneus.

4. 20 to 30% must be borne on outer weight bearing arch, and the 5th metatarsal.

5. 5 to 10% borne on the 1st metatarsal head.

6. 0% on the 2nd and 3rd metatarsal heads.

If appreciably more than 50% of the body weight is borne on one foot, the arch cannot be maintained.

If the gross weight is disproportionate to the muscle tonicity, the arches will fall.

If the heel height is such that 50% or more of the unilateral body weight shifts anterior to the intermalleolar line, the arch cannot be maintained.

If the heel height is such that 50% or more of the unilateral body weight shifts anterior to the intermalleolar line, the foot will be jammed into the toe of the shoe, regardless of the length of the shoe.

If weight bearing is assumed statically by the 2nd and 3rd metatarsal heads, metatarsalgia will be present as long as that condition persists.

If more than 10% of the unilateral body weight is assumed statically by the first metatarsal head, inversion of the arch cannot be maintained, and Hallux Valgus and bunion cannot be prevented or treated satisfactorily.

If the heel is more than 1-1/2 inches thicker than the sole, the lumbo-sacral angle will be more than 37-1/2° and the lumbar index more than 1-1/2 inches. A lumbar index of two inches or more is ALWAYS PATHOLOGICAL.

If the heel height is sufficiently low (if that can be imagined) that the lumbar index is less than one inch, that infinitely less frequent condition is similarly ALWAYS PATHOLOGICAL.

The shoe therefore has the ability to maintain good foot and super structure relations, or to destroy such mechanical requirements for the erect position.

4

FLOW OF WEIGHT
IN GOOD FOOT MECHANICS

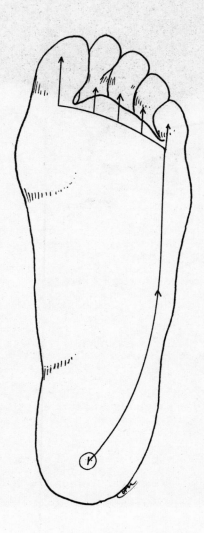

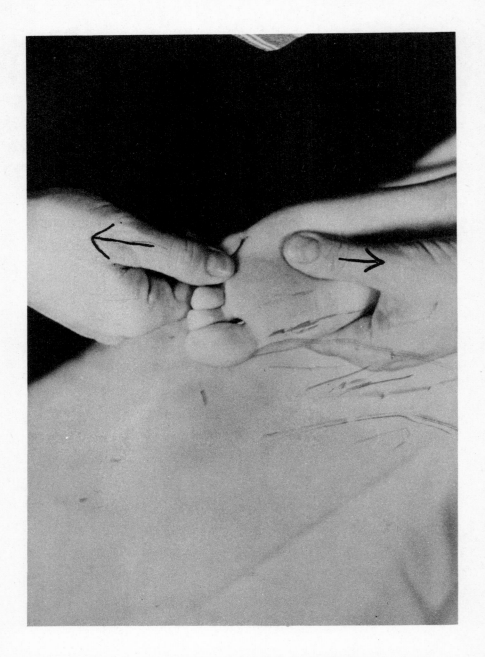

MANIPULATION TO THE PHALANGES IS PRINCIPALLY TRAC-
TION OR JOINT SEPARATION, INTERMITTENT AND RYTHM-
ICAL. SUCH MANIPULATION BREAKS FIBROUS RESTRICTION
TO MOTION AND FACILITATES RETURN CIRCULATION.

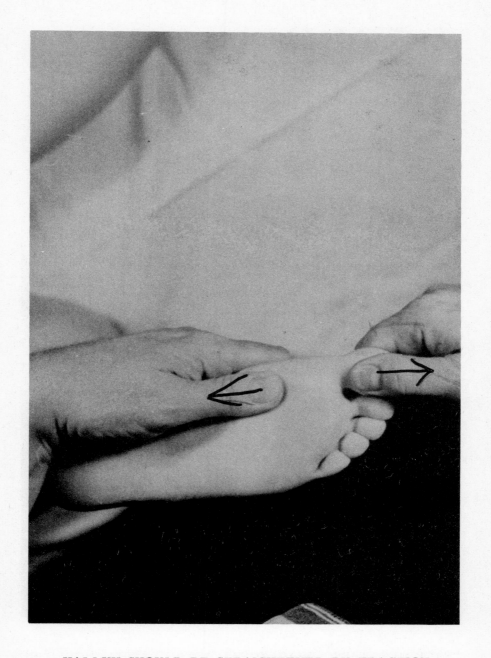

HALLUX SHOULD BE STRAIGHTENED BY TRACTION

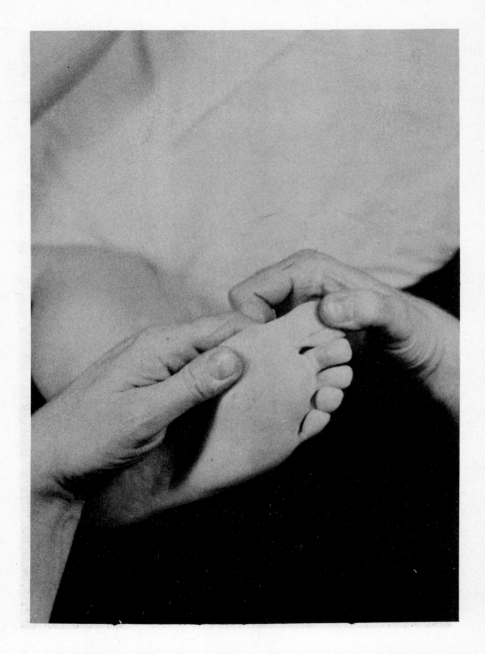

EACH METATARSO-PHALANGEAL ARTICULATION SHOULD BE
PUT THROUGH ITS COMPLETE RANGE OF MOTION.

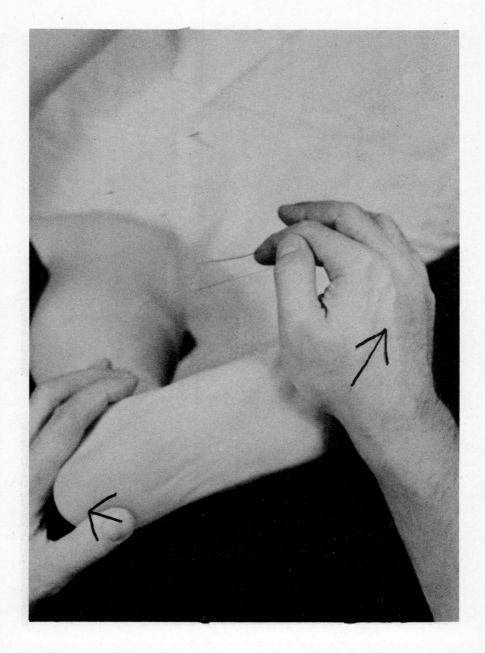

PLANTAR MUSCLE, FASCIAL, AND LIGAMENTOUS TISSUES
ARE STRETCHED TO IMPROVE RETURN CIRCULATION AND
PHYSIOLOGICAL FUNCTION.

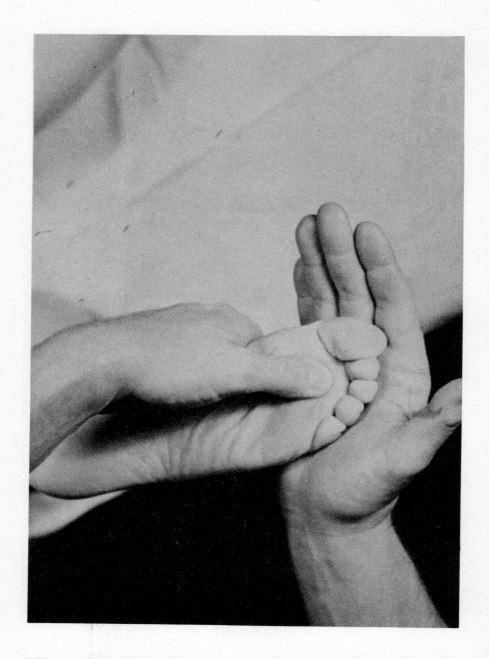

METATARSO-PHALANGEAL ARTICULATIONS MAY BE TESTED
FOR INDIVIDUAL RANGE OF MOTION IN ALL DIRECTIONS.

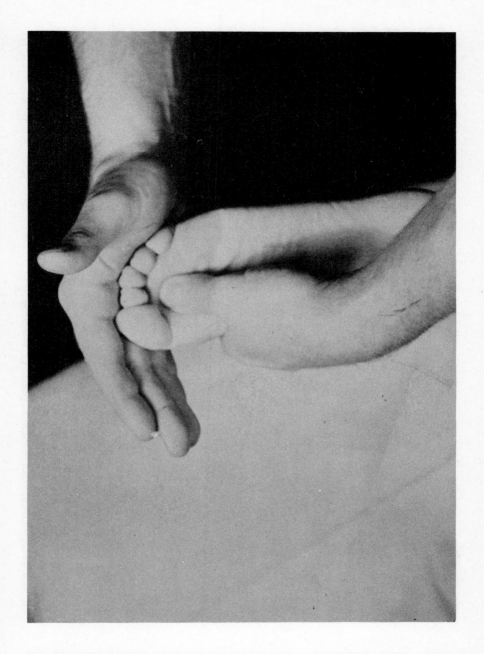

INCREASING THE RANGE OF MOTION IS MOST OFTEN NEC-
ESSARY IN THE DIRECTION OF PLANTAR FLEXION AT THE
METATARSO-PHALANGEAL ARTICULATION FOR HALLUX
FLEXUS TO HALLUX RIGIDUS.

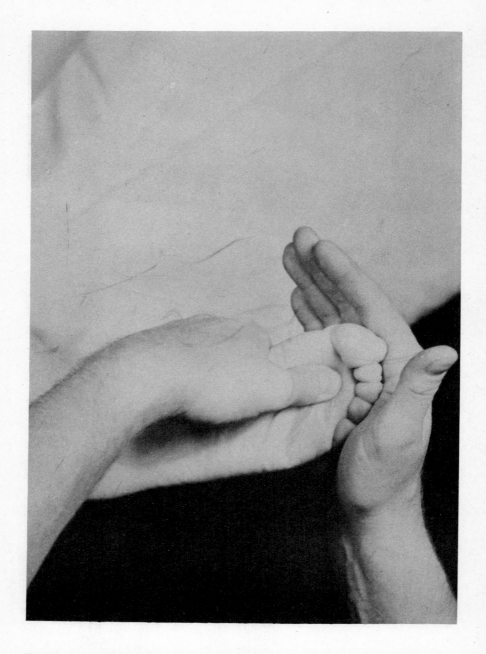

CARE IS ESSENTIAL TO PREVENT TRAUMA AND FRACTURE OF THE PHALANGES WHILE SPECIFICALLY FORCING COMPLETE MOTION. NO THRUST IS REQUIRED ORDINARILY.

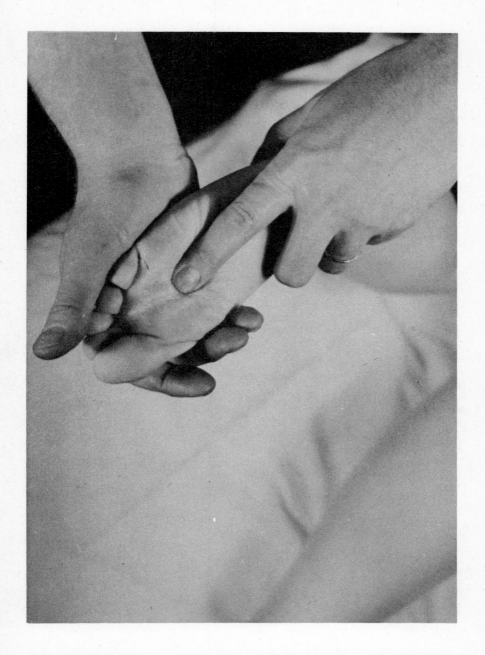

THE METATARSAL OR DISTAL END OF THE LONGITUDINAL ARCH IS CUPPED IN THE PALM OF THE HAND AND THE ARCH ELEVATED. THIS RESTORES NORMAL POSITION AND THE SHAFT OF THE METATARSAL BONES MAY BE GRASPED WITHOUT TRAUMA TO THE INTEROSSEUS TISSUES. THIS IS AN ESSENTIAL POSITION OF ALL FOOT CORRECTIONS EXCEPT IN PES CAVUS.

MANIPULATION

FOR

PES PLANUS

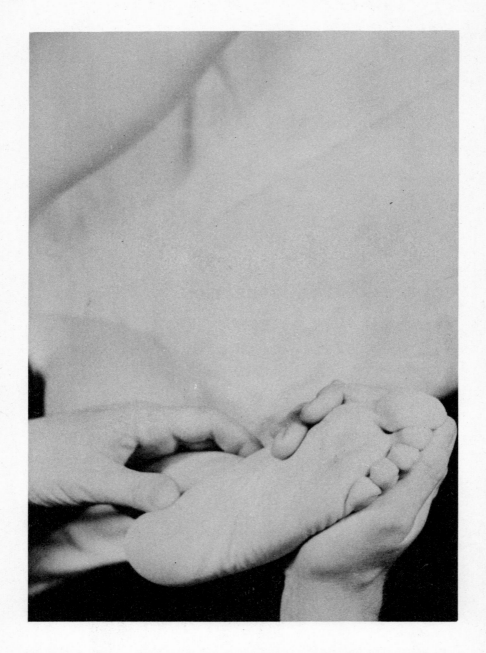

INASMUCH AS EVERY ARCH DESCENT PRODUCES EVERSION OF THE FOOT, INVERSION IS AN ESSENTIAL DIRECTION FOR CORRECTIVE POSITIONING. INVERSION SHOULD ACCOMPANY CORRECTIONAL FORCES ON ALL FEET EXCEPT PES CAVUS AND FEET CHARACTERIZED BY ABNORMAL INVERSION.

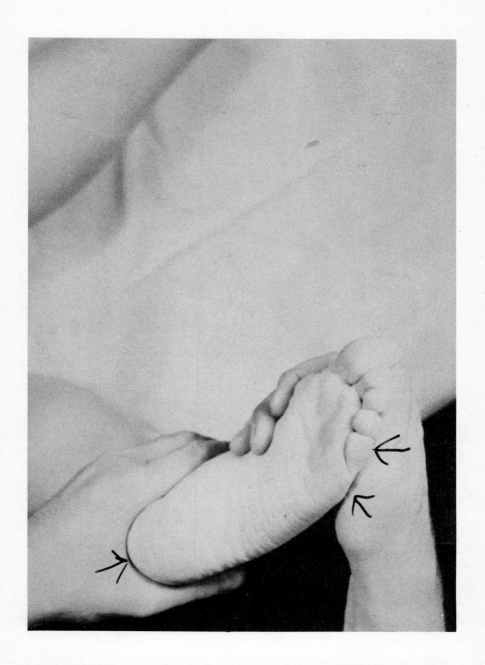

THE PLANTAR MUSCLES, FASCIAS AND LIGAMENTS ARE UN-
DER STRESS. CALCANEUS BECOMES MORE HORIZONTAL.
EACH CORRECTIVE FORCE SHOULD ACCOMPANY FOOT SHORT-
ENING TO REDUCE STRAIN ON THE ABOVE TISSUES.

THE CUNEIFORM BONES ARE WEDGE SHAPE AND ACT AS KEY-STONES IN THE LONGITUDINAL ARCH. WHEN THE ARCH FALLS THE CUNEIFORMS SPREAD, DESCEND, BECOME WEIGHT BEARING. RECONSTRUCTION OF THE ARCH REQUIRES NORMAL POSITIONING OF THE CUNEIFORM BONES.

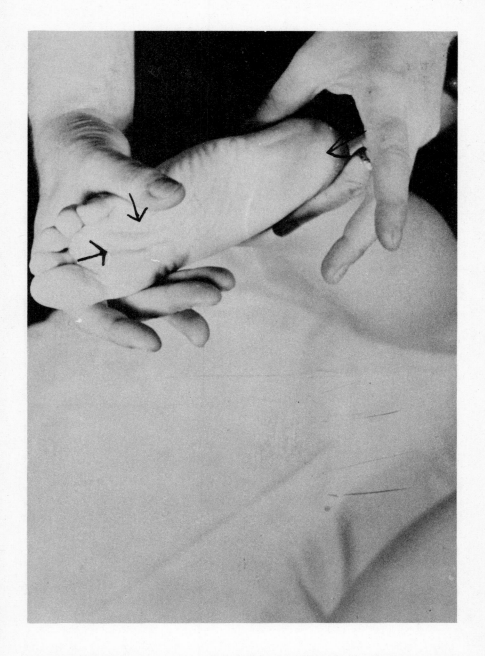

RESTORATION OF THE CUBOIDO-CUNEIFORM ARCH IS EF-
FECTED WITH THE AID OF INVERSION, ARCH ELEVATION,
AND FOOT SHORTENING MOTIONS ILLUSTRATED ABOVE,
WITH ADDITIONAL SPECIFIC FORCES ADDED.

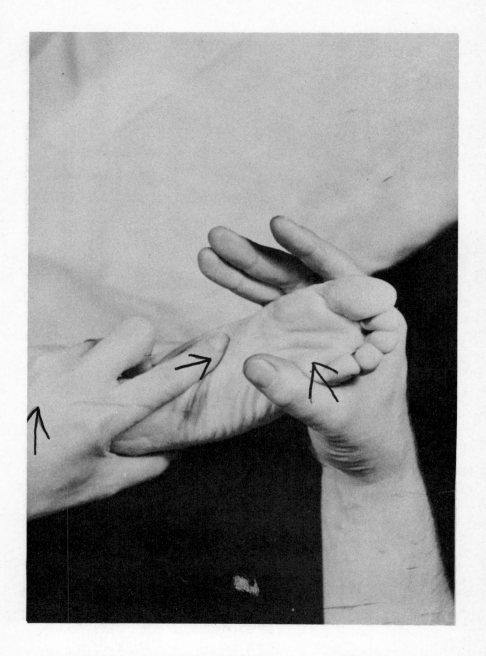

CALCANEUS IS GRASPED, AS IS THE METATARSAL SHAFT
AREA, TO INVERT AND SHORTEN FOOT. A FINGER OR TWO
IS APPLIED TO THE INFERIOR ASPECT OF THE 1ST CUNEI-
FORM.

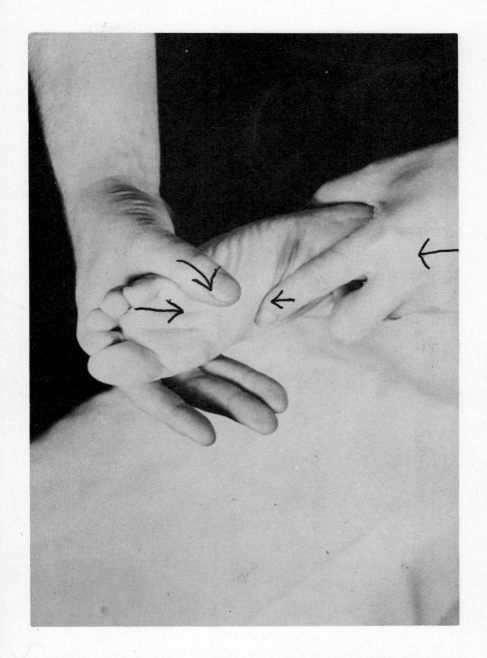

INVERSION AND PLANTAR FLEXION WITH DISTAL HAND; AND
FINGER ON PROXIMAL PORTION OF FOOT ON THE INFER-
IOR PORTION OF 1ST CUNEIFORM PRESSES UPWARD ON
PLANTAR PORTION OF CUNEIFORM TO RESTORE NORMAL
ARCH.

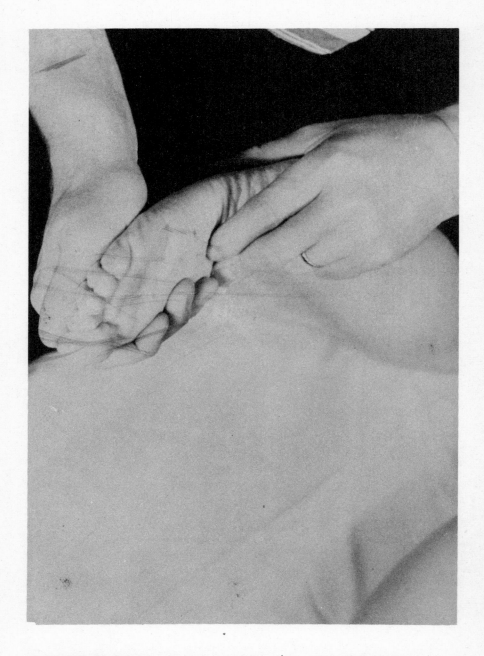

ELEVATION OF INFERIOR BORDER OF 1ST CUNEIFORM: EL-
EVATION OF SECOND ALSO.

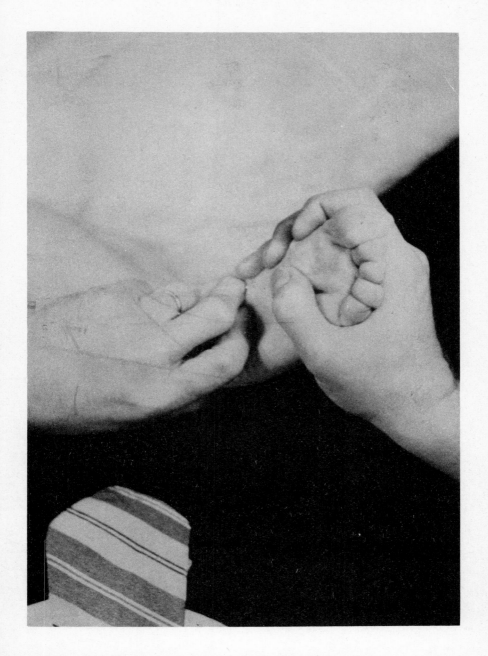

ELEVATION OF SECOND CUNEIFORM SPECIFICALLY: ELEV-
ATION OF THIRD ALSO.

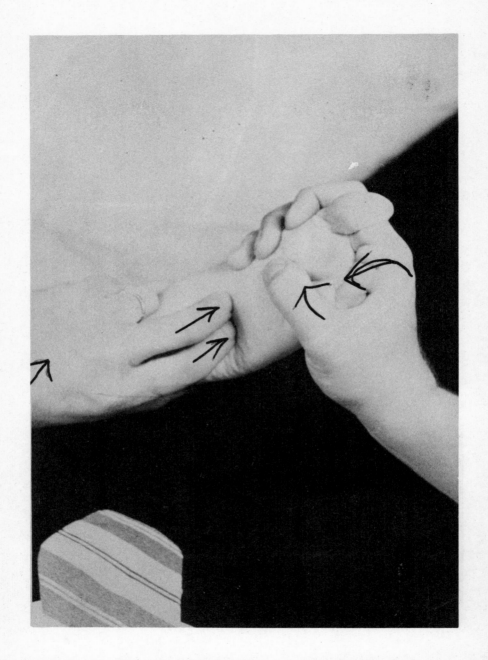

ELEVATION OF THIRD CUNEIFORM COMBINED WITH DEROTA-
TION OF THE CUBOID.

CUBOID TECHNIQUE

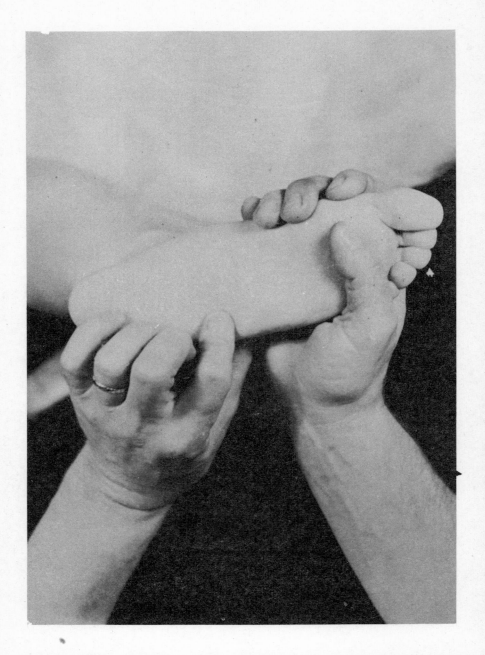

WITH EVERSION AND PES PLANUS THE CUBOID ROTATES DOWNWARD AT ITS MEDIAL MARGIN ON THE PLANTAR SURFACE.

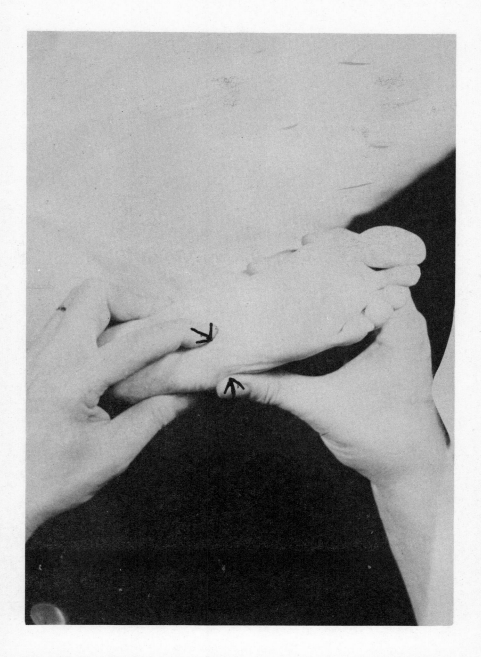

SPECIFIC CORRECTION SHOULD ELEVATE THE MEDIAL
MARGIN AND ROTATE THE CUBOID ENTIRELY.

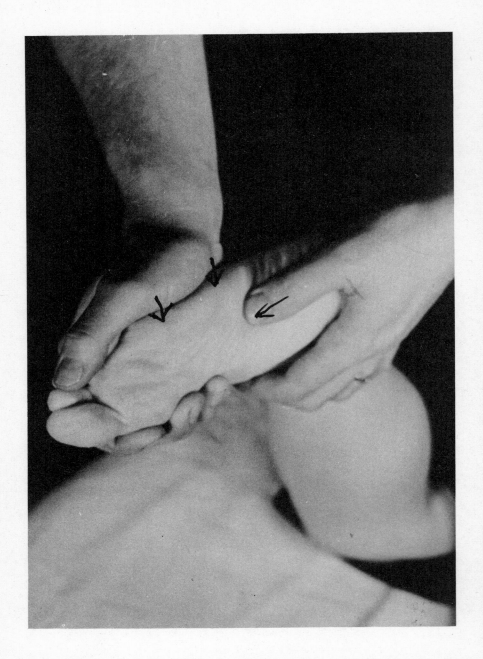

CUBOIDAL DE-ROTATION IS AIDED BY THE DISTAL HAND IN GENERAL, AND SPECIFIC CORRECTION MADE BY THUMB ON THE CUBOID. ABDUCTION OF THE LEG GIVES ADDITIONAL COUNTER FORCE.

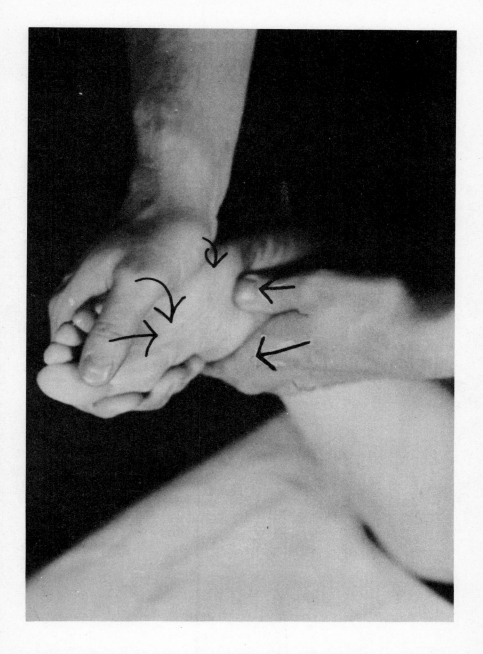

INVERSION, FOOT SHORTENING, ARCH ELEVATION AND DE-
ROTATION IS EFFECTED, WITH THE THUMB ON THE CUBOID
GIVING COUNTERFORCE ALSO.

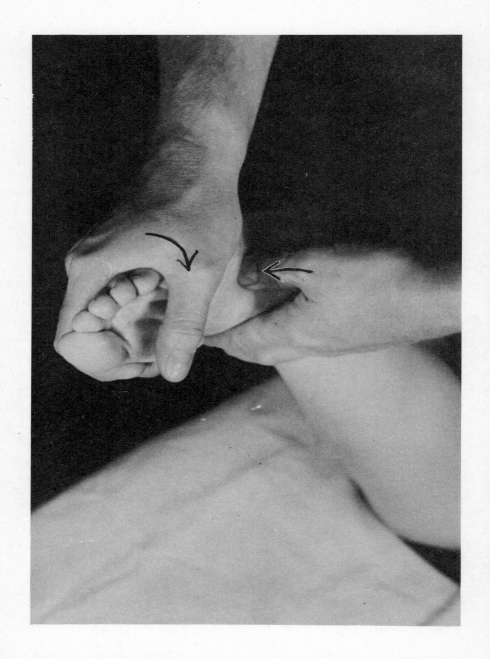

SPECIFIC CORRECTION ALONG LONG AXIS OF THUMB ELEV-
ATING THE MEDIAL BORDER OF THE CUBOID.

SNAP TECHNIQUES

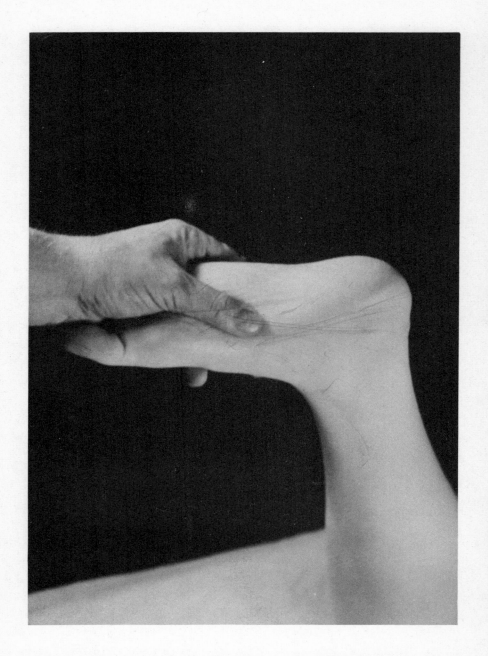

LESS SPECIFIC BUT OCCASIONALLY NECESSARY, THE "SNAP TECHNIQUE" REQUIRES A RAPID AND MORE DIFFICULTLY CONTROLLED CORRECTIVE FORCE. THUMB IS PLACED ON THE LATERAL ASPECT OF 1ST CUNEIFORM.

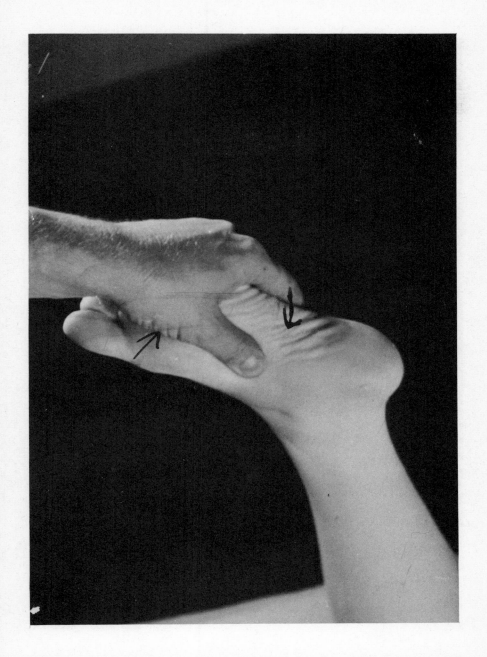

THE REST OF THE HAND GRASPS FOOT TO INVERT FOOT
AND ELEVATE ARCH.

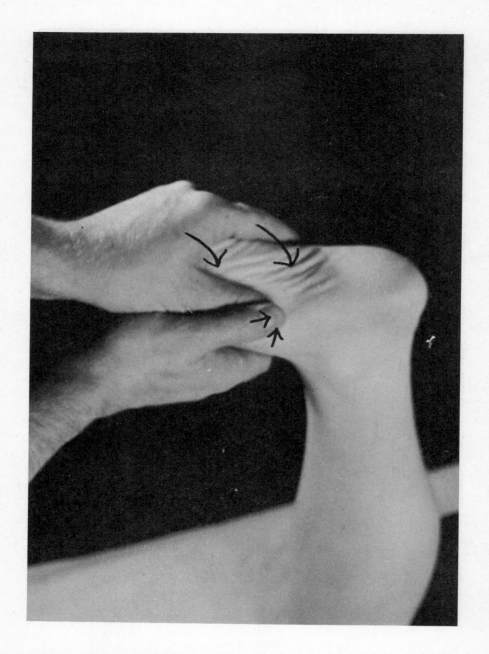

THUMB IS REINFORCED BY ITS FELLOW OVER THE BONE
TO BE SPECIFICALLY MOVED.

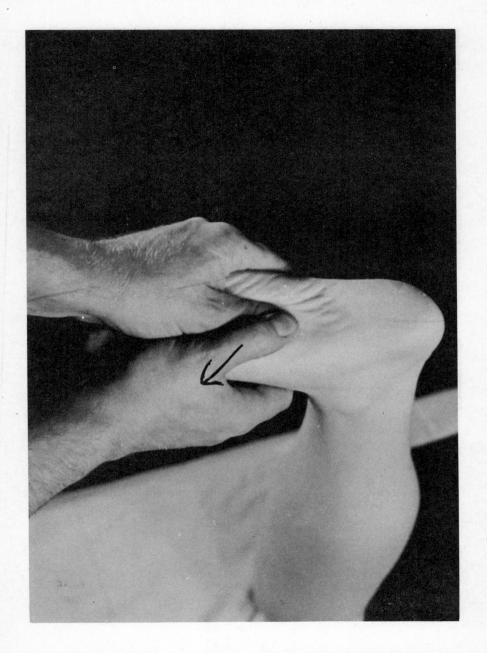

GAPPING OF ARTICULATIONS INITIATED BY EXTENSION OF
FORE-FOOT.

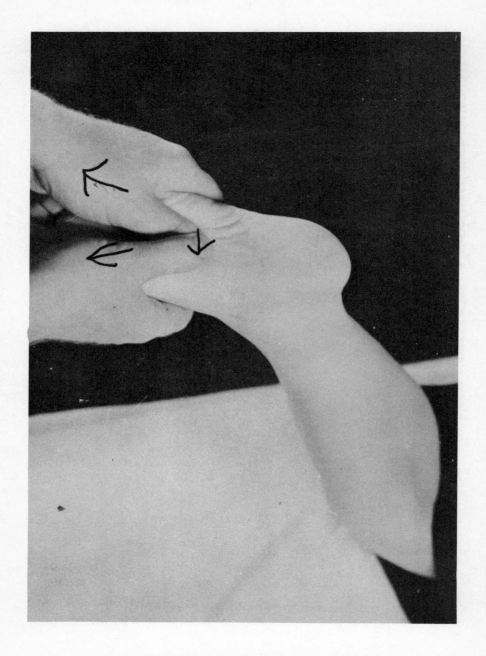

PLANTAR FLEXION STARTED ABRUPTLY.

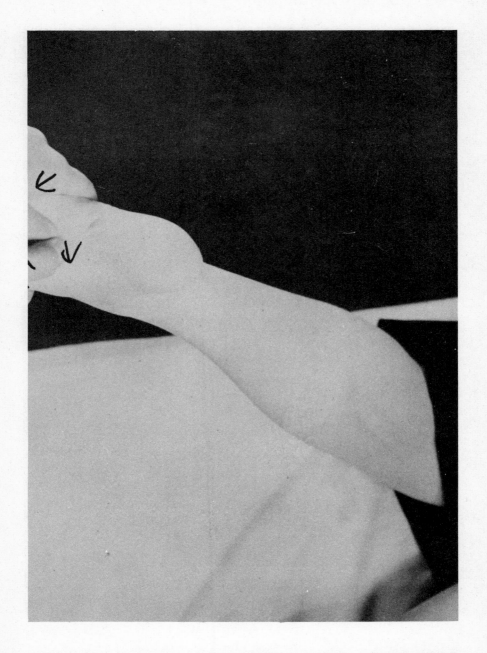

PLANTAR FLEXION AND INVERSION REACHES A SHARP PEAK
WITH THE THUMBS FORMING A FULCRUM OR THRUST POINT.

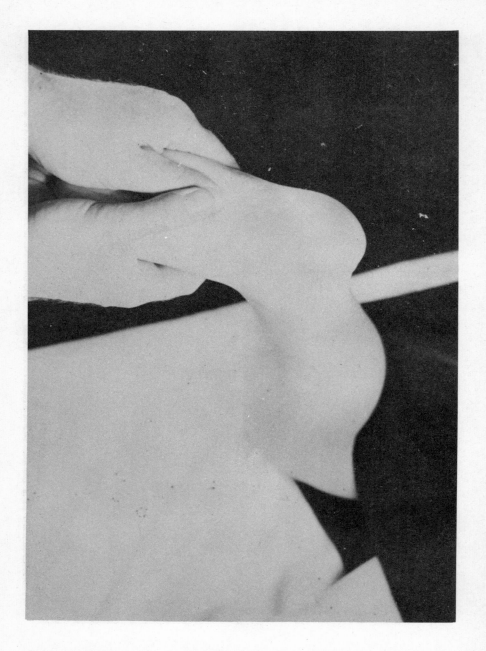

SAME "SNAP" MAY BE EXTENDED TO THE OTHER CUNEI-
FORM BONES.

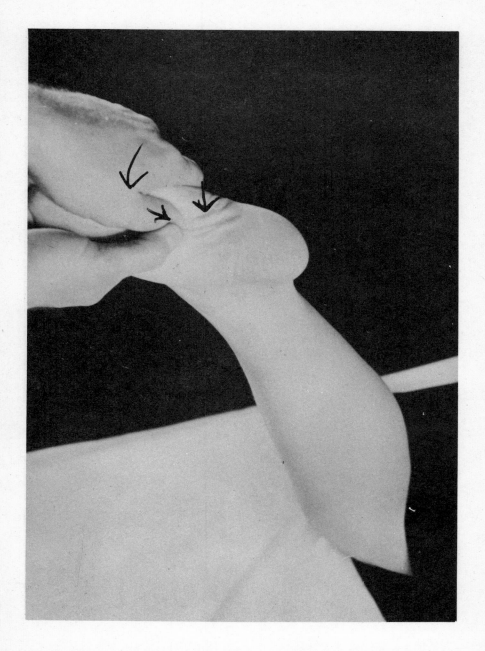

SNAP MAY BE CARRIED ONTO CUBOID. THUMBS CONTACT
MEDIAL BORDER OF THAT BONE. LATERAL HAND INVERTS
FOOT.

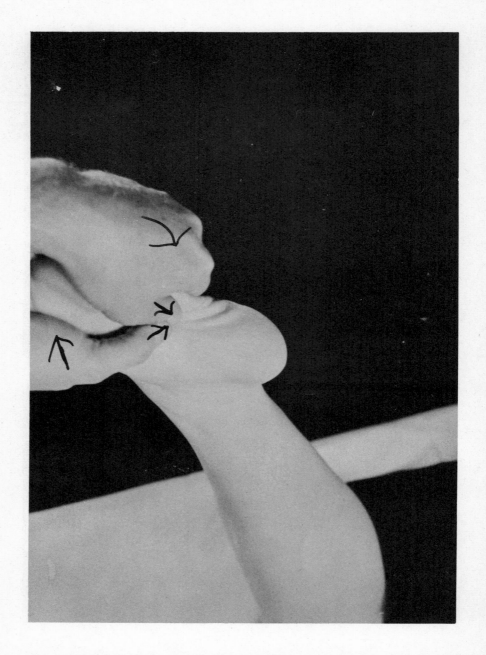

SNAP REACHES PEAK, THRUSTING MEDIAL BORDER UPWARD. LATERAL HAND FORCIBLY INVERTS FOOT AGAINST COR-RECTIVE THUMBS ON MEDIAL BORDER.

NAVICULAR TECHNIQUES

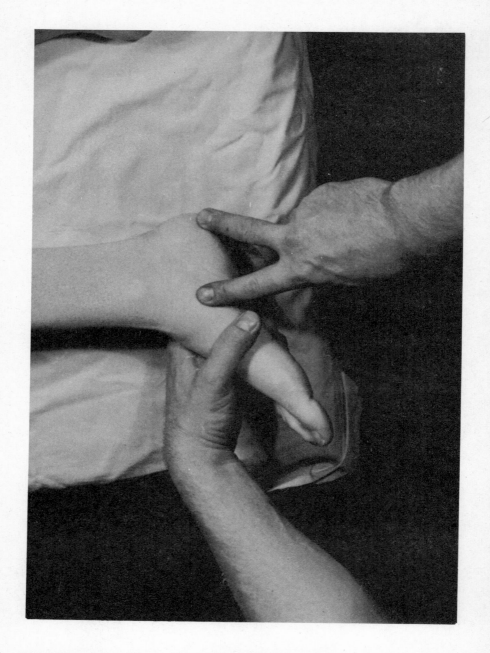

PATIENT SUPINE - NAVICULAR PROMINENCE IS THE MOST
NOTICEABLE CHARACTERISTIC OF THE EVERTED PRONATED
FOOT. THE INFERIOR PROMINENCE ROTATES UPWARD AND
THE WHOLE BONE SLIPS MEDIALLY.

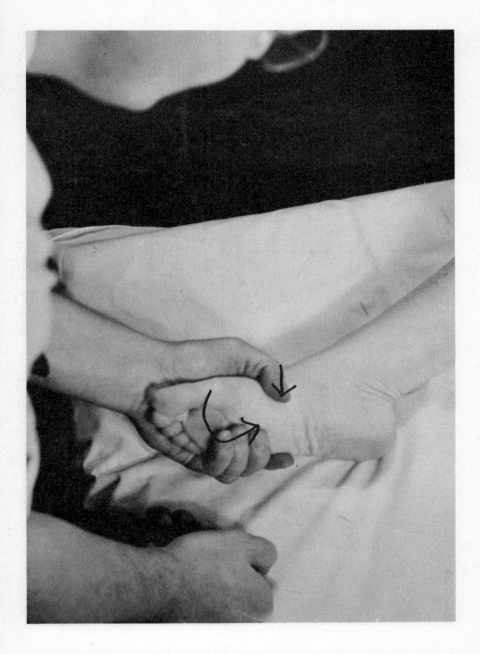

1ST CUNEIFORM IS GRASPED WITH THUMB AND FORE FOOT
INVERTED AS IN "SHAKING HANDS".

43

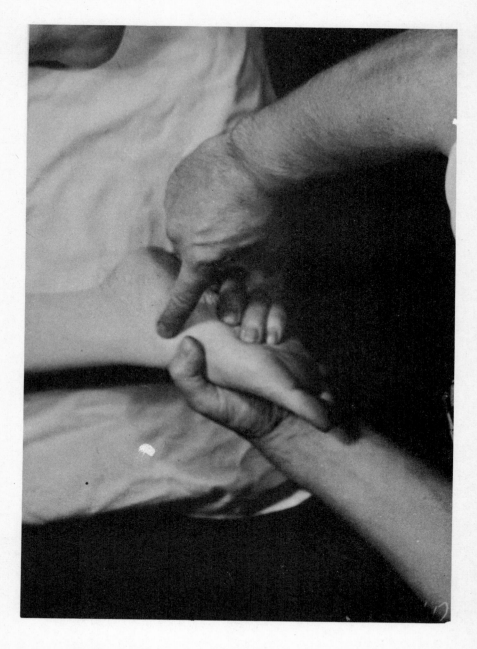

NAVICULAR EMINENCE LOCATED, CALCANEUS REMAINS ON TABLE.

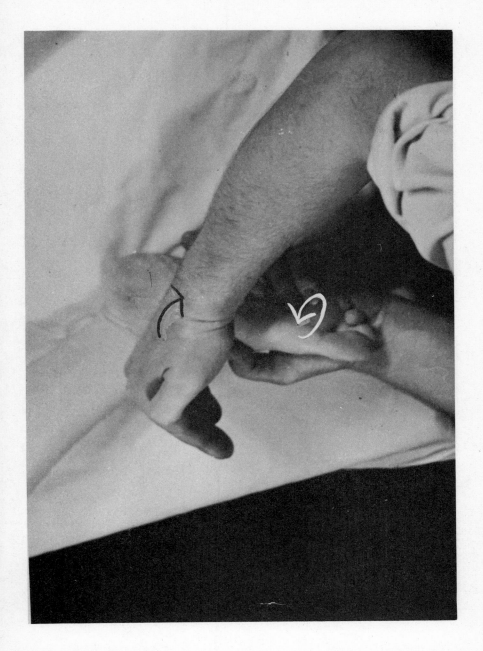

HYPOTHENAR EMINENCE PLACED ON NAVICULAR. IT IS RO-
TATED PLANTARWARD AND THRUST LATERALLY. OTHER
HAND FORCIBLY INVERTS DISTAL FOOT FOR COUNTER-
FORCE.

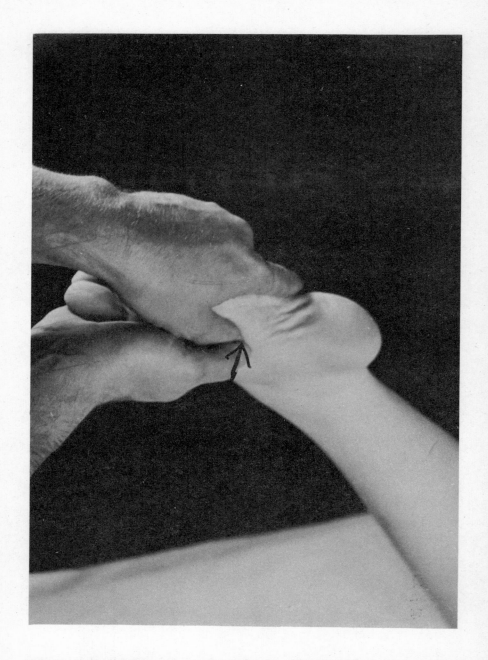

SNAP TECHNIQUE MAY BE USED- PATIENT PRONE. BOTH
THUMBS OVER THE NAVICULAR, IT IS ROTATED PLANTAR-
WARD AND THRUST LATERALLY.

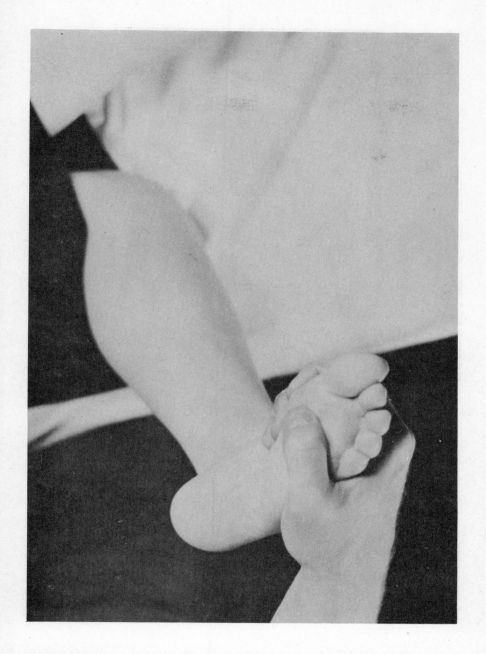

ANOTHER TWO HANDED TRACTIONAL METHOD OF DE-RO-
TATING THE NAVICULAR. THIS AND SNAP TECHNIQUE NOT
SUGGESTED. DISTAL HAND INVERTS FOOT.

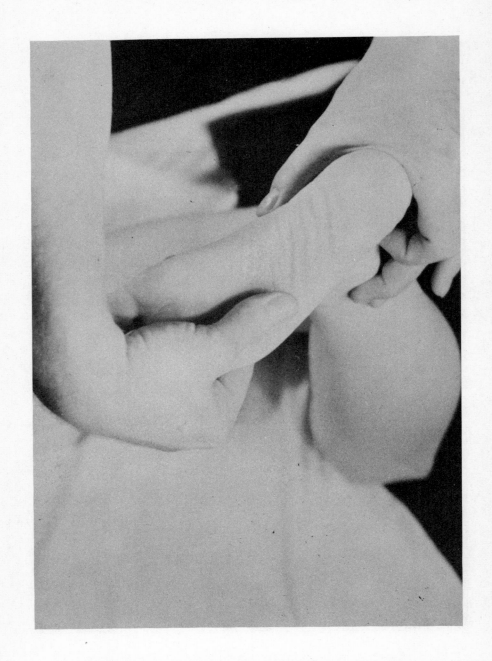

PROXIMAL HAND LOCATES NAVICULAR BONE.

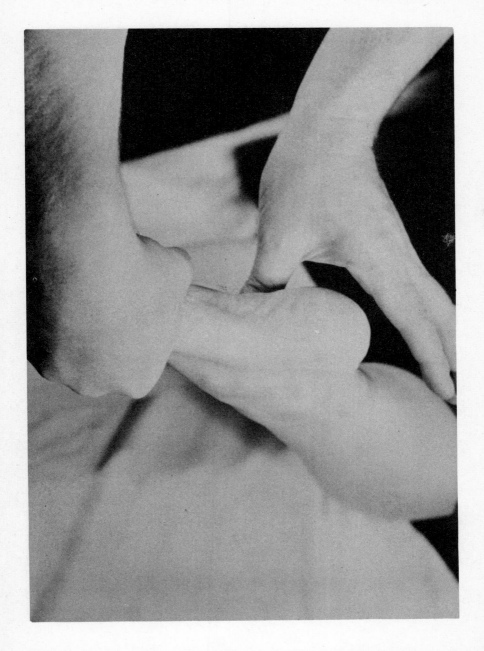

DISTAL HAND INVERTS FOOT OVER NAVICULAR CONTACT.

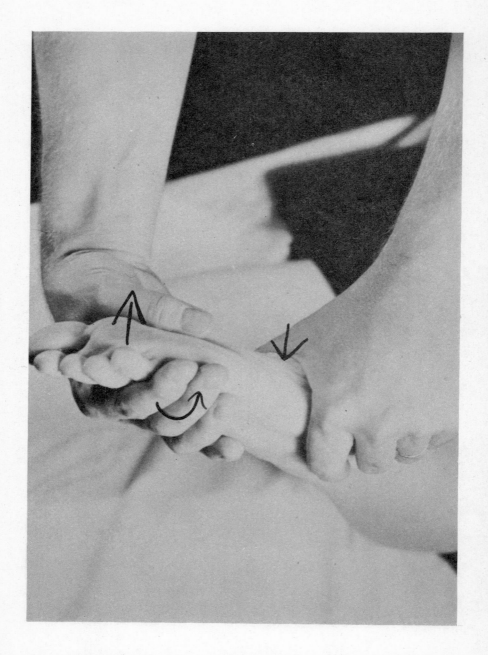

NAVICULAR IS FORCED LATERALLY, TENSION IS ACCUMU-
LATED IN INVERSION.

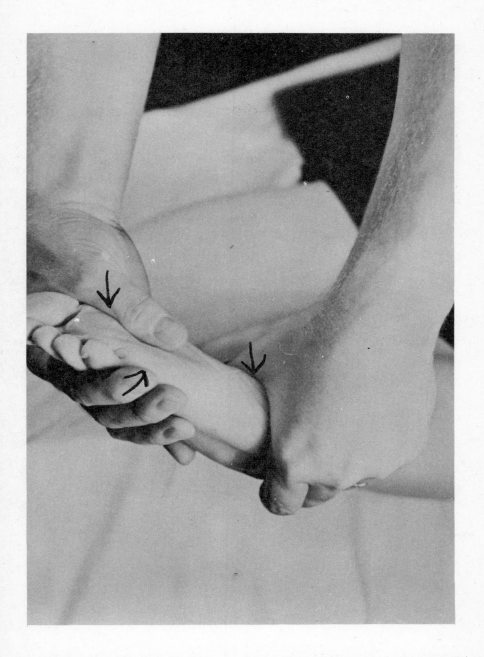

THRUST CARRIES NAVICULAR LATERALLY. FOOT HELD IN
INVERSION, ARCH ELEVATION, AND FOOT SHORTENED.

TALUS TECHNIQUES

IN PES PLANUS THE SUPERIOR ARTICULAR SURFACE OF THE TALUS TILTS MEDIALLY AND INFERIORLY. TIBIA TENDS TO GRAVITATE MEDIALLY, IMPINGING THE FIBULAR MALLEOLUS AGAINST THE LATERAL ASPECT OF THE TALUS. THE FOLLOWING ARE TECHNIQUES FOR CORRECTION.

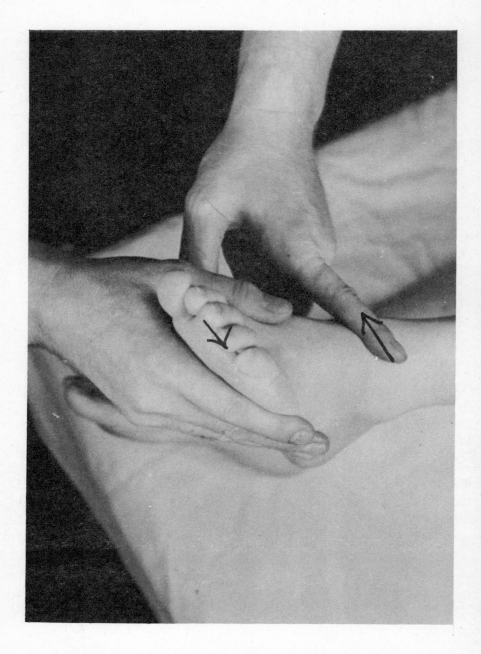

SUPERIOR ASPECT OF TALUS TILTS MEDIALLY AND DOWN-
WARD AS FOOT EVERTS. TIBIA SLIPS DOWNWARD ON THE
TILTING TALUS IMPINGING THE MALLEOLUS OF THE FIBULA.

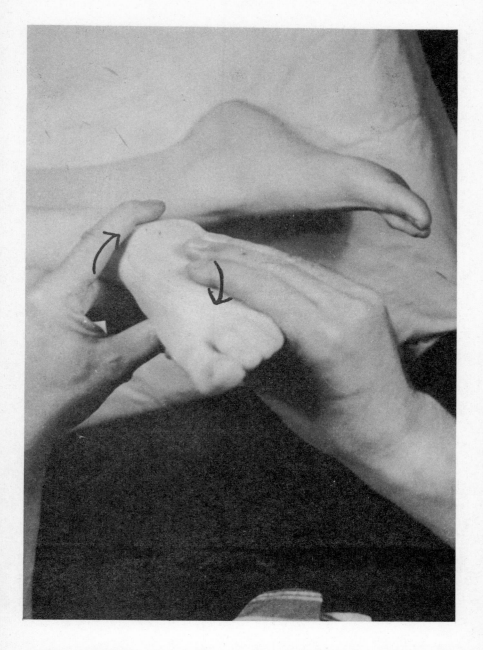

TALUS SHOULD BE PULLED INTO INVERSION AND AWAY
FROM FIBULA.

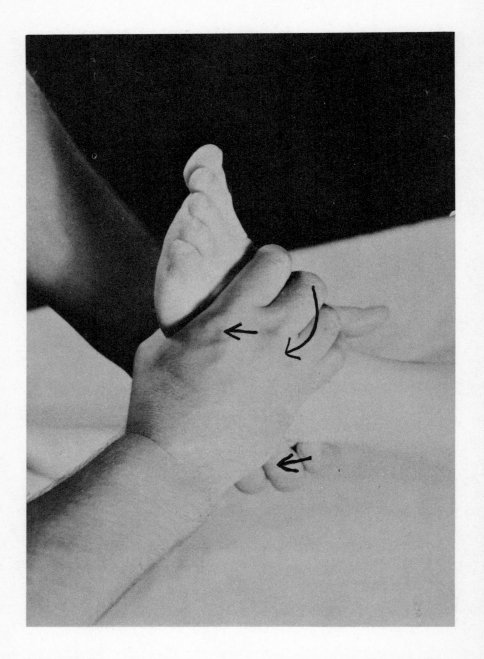

INVERSION OF FOOT AND TALUS CULMINATING IN TRACTION
SEPARATION.

CALCANEUS TECHNIQUES

PES PLANUS FINDS THE CALCANEUS FLATTENED TO A MORE HORIZONTAL POSITION WITH INCREASED TENSION ON PLANTAR MUSCLES, FASCIAS, AND LIGAMENTS.

THE CALCANEUS MUST BEAR 60 - 70% OF THE UNILATERAL BODY WEIGHT. UNLESS THE CALCANEUS IS IN NORMAL PO-SITION AND HELD BY NORMAL MUSCLE TONICITY, FOOT FUNCTION CAN NOT BE PHYSIOLOGICAL.

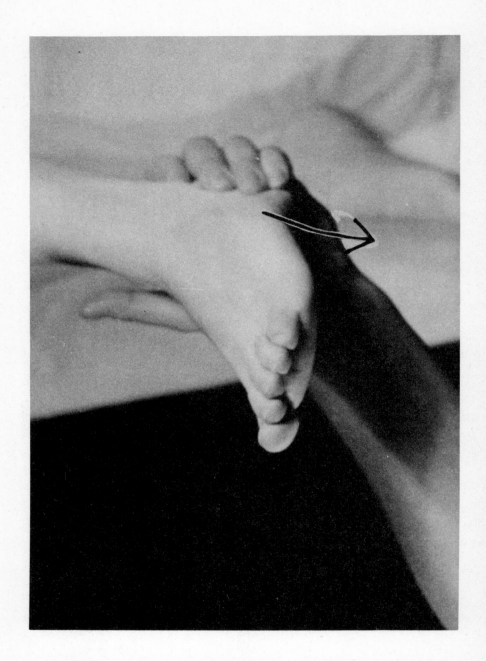

CALCANEUS ASSUMES AN ABNORMALLY HORIZONTAL PLANE.
HANDS GRASPING THE POSTERIOR ASPECT AND PULLING IT
DOWNWARD PERMITS A MORE VERTICAL LONGITUDINAL
AXIS AND BETTER WEIGHT ASSUMPTION.

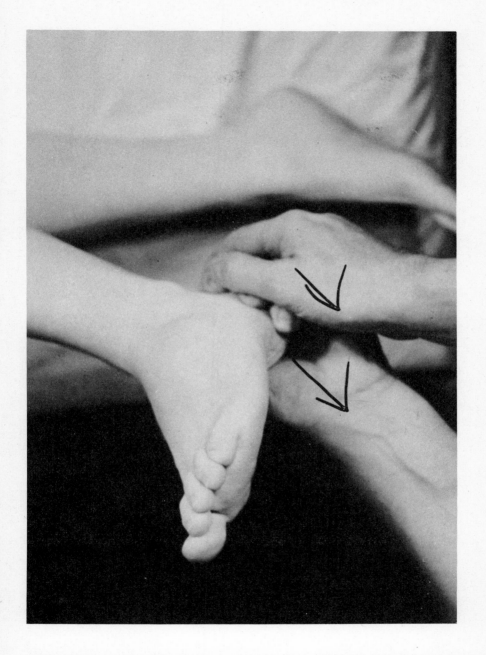

TRACTION MAY BE APPLIED TO CALCANEUS WITH BOTH HANDS.

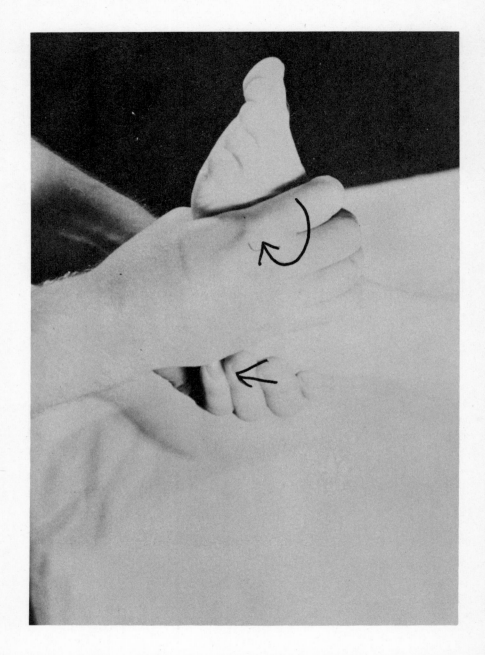

TRACTIONAL CORRECTION OF BOTH TALUS AND CALCANEUS
MAY BE APPLIED COINCIDENTLY. PROXIMAL HAND GIVES
STRAIGHT TRACTION ON CALCANEUS. DISTAL HAND GIVES
INVERSION AND TRACTION SEPARATION ON TALUS.

KNEE AREA

ANATOMICAL RELATIONS

An imaginary line from the anterior superior iliac spine to the middle of the great toe should bisect the patella, run over the patellar tendon, tibial tuberosity and descend on the rest of the tibial shaft for three to four inches.

The margins of femur and tibia at their articulation should form a smooth symmetrical apposition without marked prominence of either bone on either side.

Cruciate ligaments prevent rotation only when the leg is extended fully on the femur, hence the danger of injury in partial flexion.

The collateral ligaments should prevent gapping of joints in adduction or abduction of leg on femur.

The commonest pathology is lateral tibial torsion.

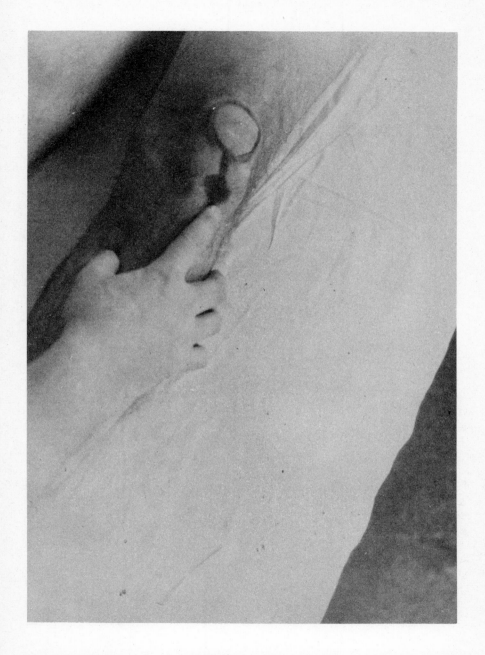

PALPATION OF ANATOMICAL RELATIONS IN KNEE AREA

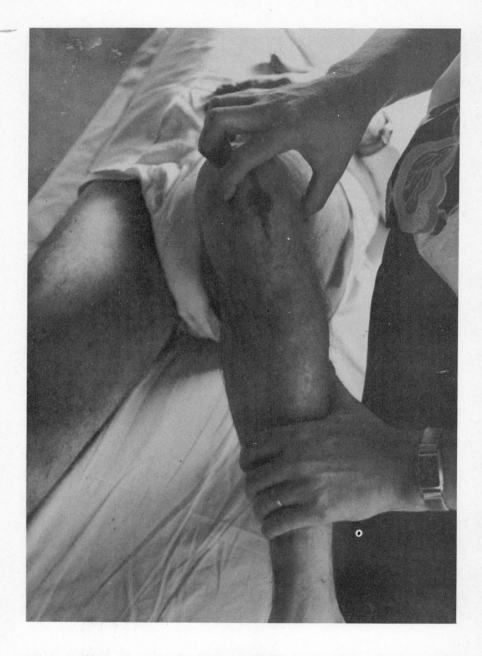

PALPATION OF MOTION AND RELATIONS IN KNEE AREA
CONTACTING MEDIAL MENISCUS AND FIBULA.

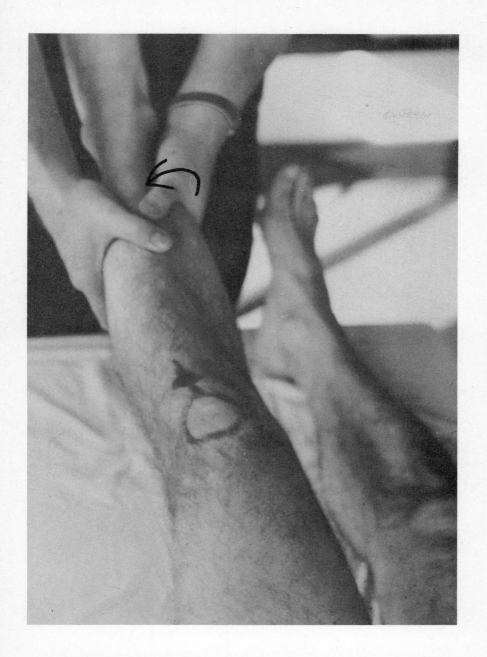

SEPARATION AND ROTATION OF KNEE JOINT. ALSO LATERAL
FLEXION TO DETERMINE LIGAMENTOUS SUPPORT.

LATERAL TIBIAL TORSION

External rotation is the most frequent malalignment in the knee. It is present in every pes planus, weight shift laterally or ventrally, and may be acquired thru trauma.

Diagnosis: Medial proximal portion of tibia is anterior and prominent, lateral portion of tibia is posterior and less prominent than femur, and patellar tendon deviates laterally toward the laterally rotated patellar or tibial tuberosity. Crest of tibia is lateral also to the anatomical line.

There will be pain and hypertonicity around the fibular head and in the biceps femoris muscle.

Pain more acute over medial anterior and lateral posterior aspects of knee joint.

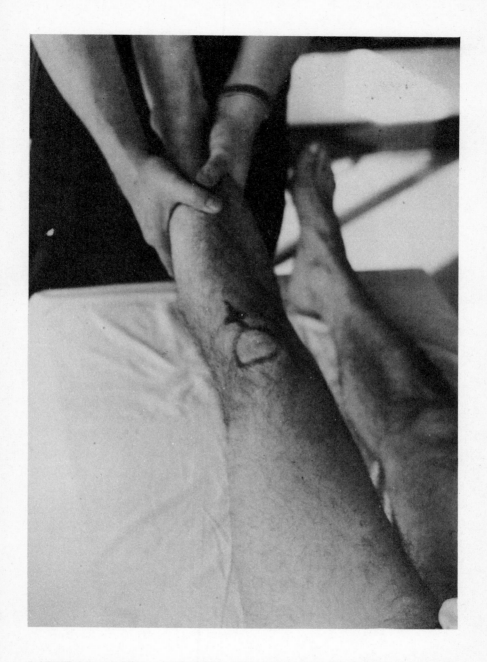

LATERAL TIBIAL TORSION CORRECTED AS CONDITION RE-
QUIRES WITH OR WITHOUT LOCAL OR GENERAL ANESTHESIA.
GRASPING SHAFT OF TIBIA - STRAIGHT TRACTION IS APPLIED
FIRST.

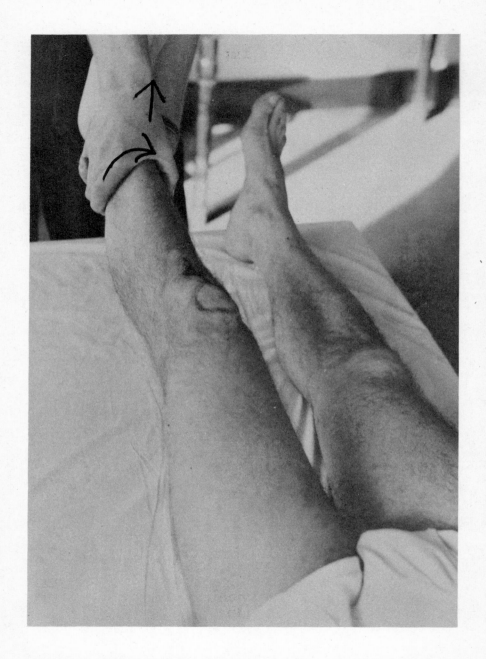

WHILE TRACTION IS MAINTAINED INTERNAL OR MEDIAL RO-
TATION IS PRODUCED. FIBROUS RESTRICTIONS WILL BE
FELT BREAKING AS THE TIBIA IS NUDGED STRONGLY. THIS
IS PROBABLY THE TECHNIQUE OF CHOICE IN ACUTE KNEES,
FRACTURED MENISCUS AND IN RARE INSTANCES SLIPPED
MENISCUS.

PROXIMAL FIBULA

FIBULAR CONSIDERATIONS

The proximal end of the fibula is frequently involved with a lateral tibial torsion. The fibula is rotated posteriorly and the biceps femoris muscle attaching to it and the knee joint capsule will maintain the posterior head and the lateral tibial torsion.

Posterior fibular head is present in every pes planus; every weight shift laterally or ventrally, and is acquired also by trauma.

While lateral tibial torsion and posterior fibular head are present, the knee joint is under constant chronic sprain and soft tissue strain.

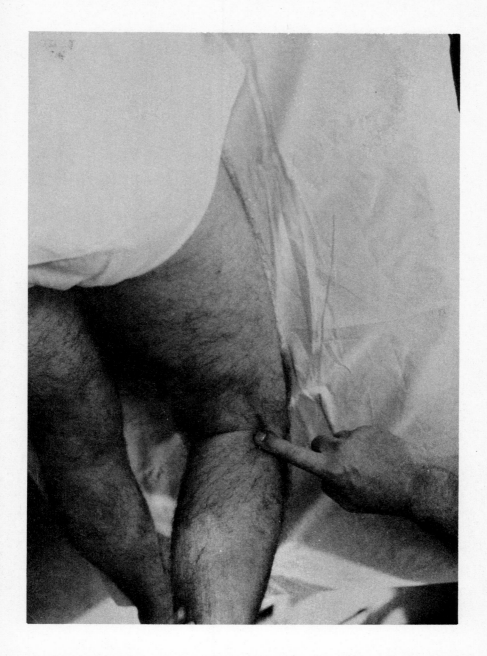

PATIENT PRONE - TECHNIQUE FOR LATERAL TIBIAL TOR-
SION OR POSTERIOR FIBULAR HEAD OR BOTH. POSTERIOR
ASPECT OF LATERAL TIBIAL AND/OR FIBULA LOCATED.

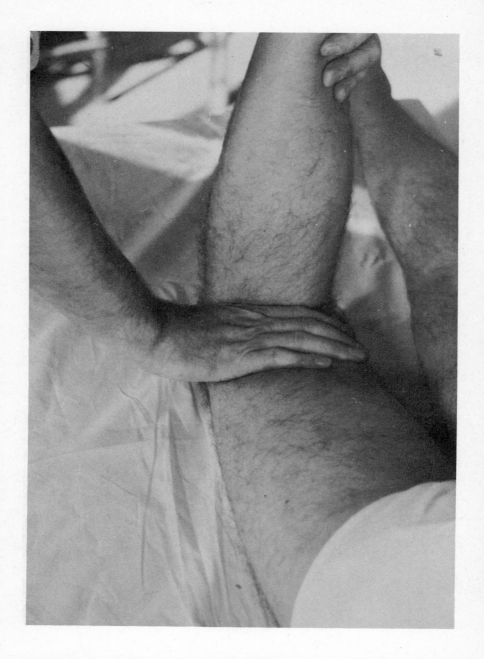

HAND AS A WEDGE, THICKER PORTION LATERALLY AGAINST
POSTERIOR FIBULAR HEAD.

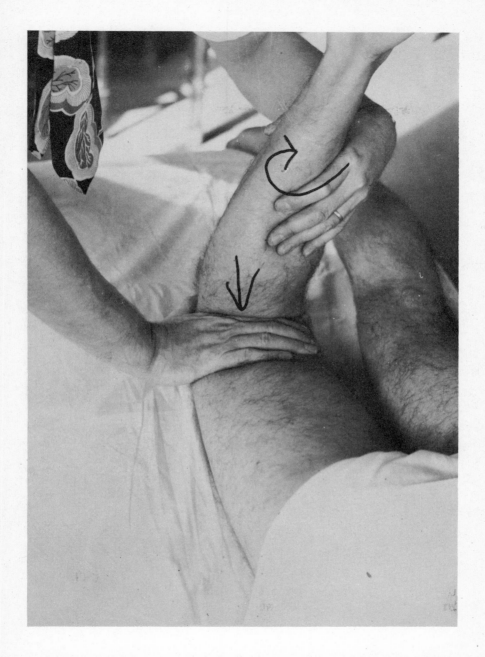

LEG IS INTERNALLY ROTATED AND FLEXED OVER HAND IN POPLITEAL SPACE.

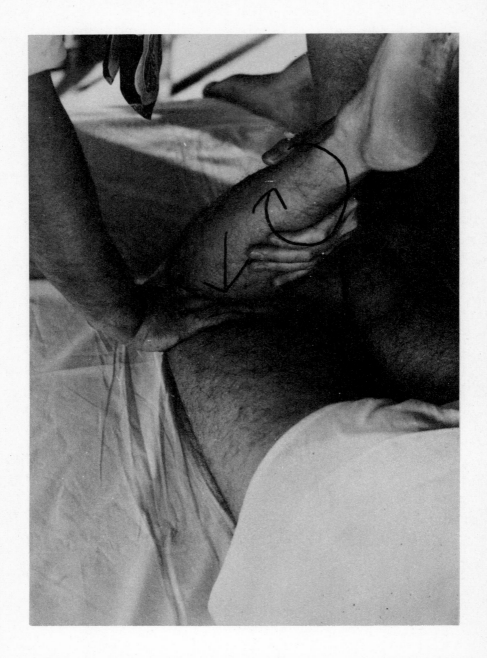

FORCED INTERNAL ROTATION OF TIBIA AND PRESSURE OF
HAND MAGNIFIED BY COMPLETE FLEXION COMPRESSING
POSTERIOR FIBULA AND TIBIA, AND CARRYING THEM AN-
TERIORLY.

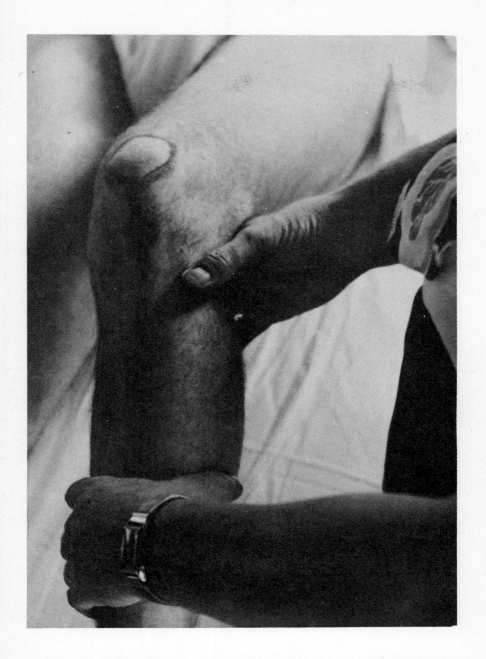

SIMILAR TECHNIQUE - PATIENT SUPINE. HAND AS WEDGE, PLACED IN PREVIOUS POSITION. FORCED INTERNAL TIBIAL ROTATION AND HYPERFLEXION OVER WEDGE FORCES TIBIA AND FIBULA ANTERIORLY.

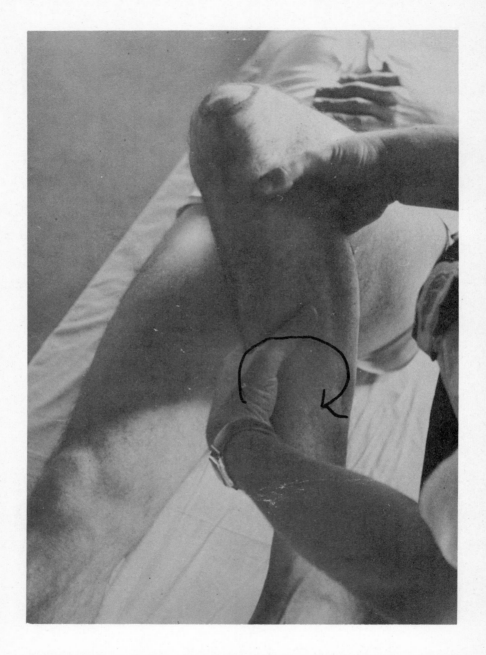

SIMILAR TECHNIQUE - PATIENT SUPINE. HAND AS WEDGE, PLACED IN PREVIOUS POSITION. FORCED INTERNAL TIBIAL ROTATION AND HYPERFLEXION OVER WEDGE FORCES TIBIA AND FIBULA ANTERIORLY.

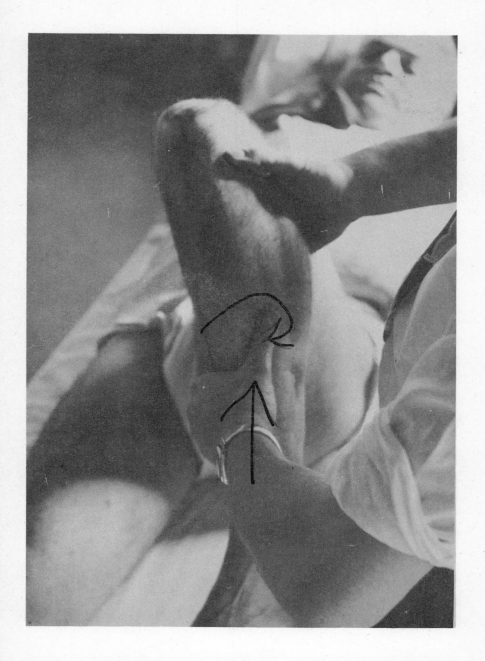

SIMILAR TECHNIQUE - PATIENT SUPINE. HAND AS WEDGE, PLACED IN PREVIOUS POSITION. FORCED INTERNAL TIBIAL ROTATION AND HYPERFLEXION OVER WEDGE FORCES TIBIA AND FIBULA ANTERIORLY.

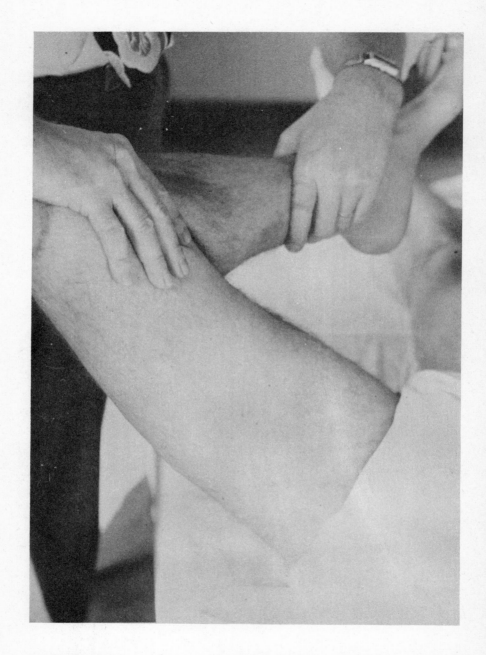

MODIFICATION FOR A MEDIAL TIBIAL TORSION. THUMB
PLACED MEDIALLY AND POSTERIORLY. FLEXION ROTATES
TIBIA LATERALLY - UNUSUAL TRAUMATIC CONDITION.

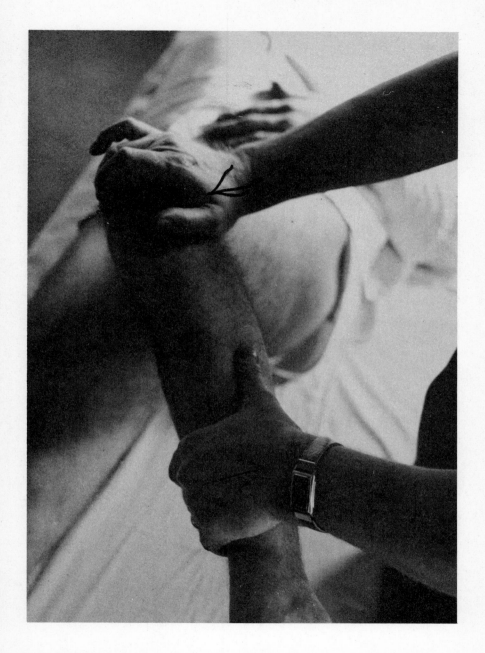

TECHNIQUE FOR SLIPPED CARTILAGE AND/OR LATERAL
TIBIAL TORSION. JOINT IS MEDIALLY GAPPED BY ABDUC-
TION ON THE DISTAL LEG OVER THE PROXIMAL HAND.
PRESSURE AND INTERNAL ROTATION BY PROXIMAL HAND
ON MEDIAL MENISCUS AND UPPER TIBIA.

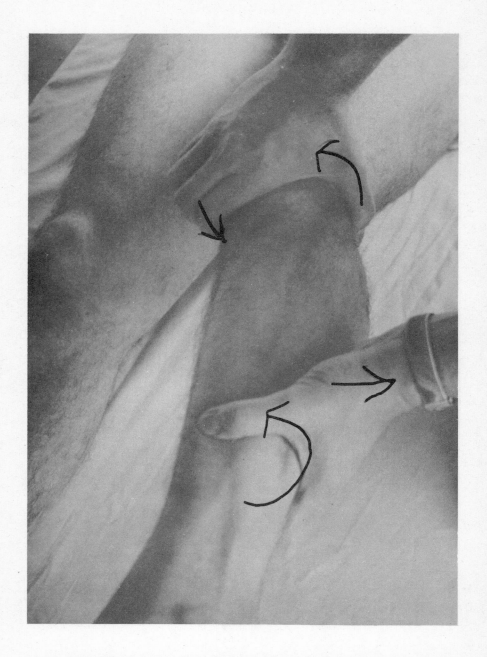

ABOVE PRESSURES AND FORCES HELD, WHILE DISTAL HAND
AIDS AND IN SAME MOTION STRAIGHTENS LEG ON FEMUR.

HIP JOINT AREA

LEG LENGTH DIFFERENCE

78 to 80% of all people have actual leg length differences. 52% of the shortness is on the left side. The average difference is 1 cm. The greater the difference, the greater the locomotive error and chronic postural trauma. We have found two cases of congenital leg length difference of three full inches.

Most differences are congenital in etiology; however a leg may be shortened or lengthened by fracture. Shortness may also be due to coxa vera, epiphyseal closure due to trauma or infection or arrest of growth due to trauma, neuritis, poliomyelitis etc. The final in measurement is standing pelvic X-ray. All leg length difference must be compensated for in the erect position.

COMPENSATION MECHANICS

The weight shifts disproportionately toward the long leg side. The long leg carries more weight and strikes the ground harder, resulting in that ilium being rocked posteriorly, giving a flexed lower sacrum on that side, which diminishes the sacral tilt. The other ilium is pulled forward in this compensation process, which leaves that side of the sacrum postero-superiorly placed in extension, elevating the sacral top on the short leg side. Therefore a sacral torsion toward the short leg side is called a compensatory sacral torsion and tends to level the sacral top. It should not be corrected until the leg lengths are equalized by adequate lift therapy.

Approximately 50% of those having leg length differences compensate completely by sacral torsion and have no scoliosis. These people develop no trouble unless they traumatically lose the compensatory torsion that protects the lumbar spine. The remaining 50% of those having different leg lengths have scoliotic tension stresses or compensatory scolioses. In this group the difference may be in excess of the 1/4 inch for which the sacrum may compensate by torsion; or there may be no compensation by the sacrum, which throws the lumbar spine to the side of the short extremity in direct relation to the difference in support given by the femoral heads.

The patient may traumatically acquire a sacral torsion to the long leg side. This further unlevels the sacral top 1/4 inch which is added to the leg length difference, exaggerating the lateral thrust thrown into the spinal area.

An unlevel sacral top due to torsion or leg length difference or both is usually compensated by the development of scoliosis. The first lumbar curve is usually convex to the side of the low sacrum. More frequently there are three curves in this compensatory pattern: lumbar and cervical convex to the low sacral side, and thoracic convex toward the opposite side.

70% of all scolioses are secondary or compensatory and should be grossly improved in those under 50 and favorably aided in those above 50.

MANAGEMENT OF LEG LENGTH DIFFERENCE

Treatment of this condition entails the placing of adequate lift to obtain either level femoral heads or a level top in corrected sacro-iliac relations with no scoliosis above.

Age will vary this routine. In a growing youngster over correction may be applied to markedly overwork the anatomically short extremity and thereby force it to grow faster. Over a period of time the short leg may be managed so that at the time of epiphyseal closure there will be no disparity between the two sides and no compensatory changes residual.

Lift therapy, when the epiphyses are closed, will stop with either level femoral heads, or a level corrected sacral top without scoliosis. In older folks, those above 50, usually the level sacrum is the index.

Lift of 1/4 inch may be placed at once in those under 50. For those patients above 50 1/8 inch lift is adequate at first insertion.

Subsequent lifts of 1/8 inch may be added, if needed, at 2 or 3 week intervals until the necessary amount is inserted.

All the lift in excess of 1/2 inch should go into the sole also.

GENERAL CONSIDERATIONS

Simple inflammatory processes in the hip joint are rare, probably due to its great range of motion.

Pain and muscle spasm splinting the hip joint is usually indicative of serious joint disease. Metastatic lesions are most common in the hip joint, probably due to the anatomical pull of the ligaments and capsule in assuming the erect position.

Hence, generous use of X-ray for diagnosis when true hip joint pain is present is mandatory.

In a patient giving a history of trauma, X-ray should be used.

With a history of removal of a tumor or operation of undisclosed cause in a patient developing true hip joint pain within five years, always X-ray.

Hip joint disease is simulated by periarticular structures. These must be isolated before mobilization in this area.

ANTERIOR HIP AREA PAIN

Psoasitis is the commonest cause, and it may be produced reflexly by at least eighteen abdominal pelvic and spinal factors.

Treatment of psoasitis and psoas fibrositis will necessitate the correction of whichever of those eighteen factors is involved. In addition stretching and relaxing by traction, diathermy, segmental blocks etc. may be necessary.

POSTERIOR AREA PAIN AND MYOSITIS

Pain in this area, when not due to the infrequent hip joint disease, is usually due to sacro-iliac strains or lesions, sciatic neuritis, and posterior myositis. Pelvic or lower abdominal reflex disturbance is always suspected and investigated.

Treatment requires the correction of the etiological factor along with local treatment. Local treatment may include diathermy, procainizations, calcium gluconate intravenously, and stretching of the external rotators by internal rotation of femur. Stretching of the hamstring musculature by straight leg raising may also be necessary.

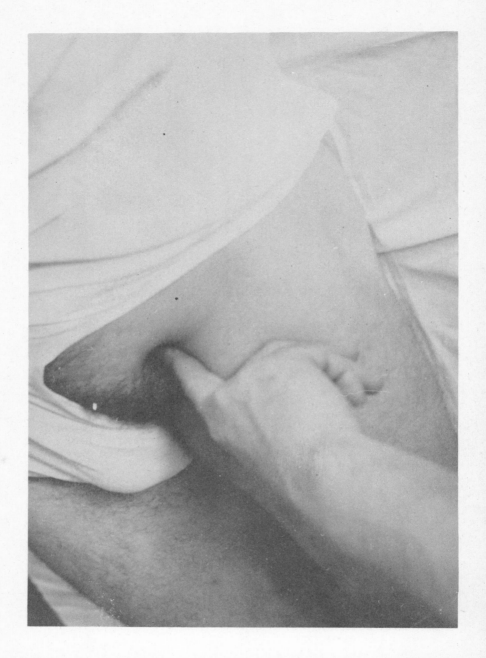

SIMULATED HIP JOINT DISEASES, PSOAS AND ILIACUS TENDO-
SYNOVITIS. COMBINED MUSCLE LEAVES PELVIS UNDER IN-
GUINAL LIGAMENT, PASSES IMMEDIATELY IN FRONT OF HIP
JOINT TO ATTACH AT LESSER FEMORAL TUBEROSITY.

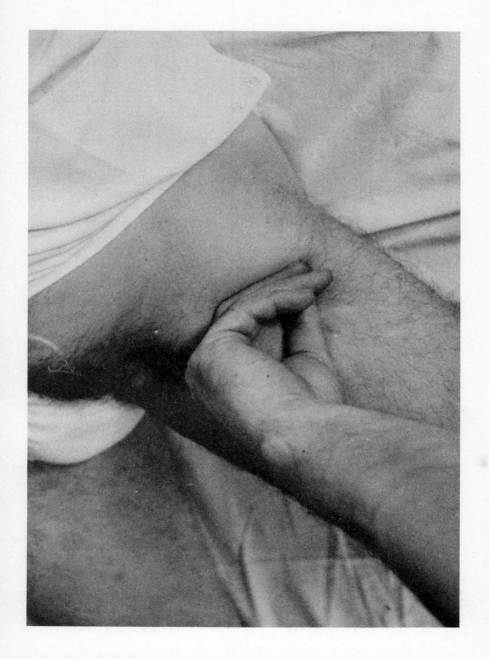

TENDERNESS WILL BE ELICITED IN EACH OF THESE AREAS
AS WELL AS THE VERTEBRAL AND ILIAL ORIGIN.

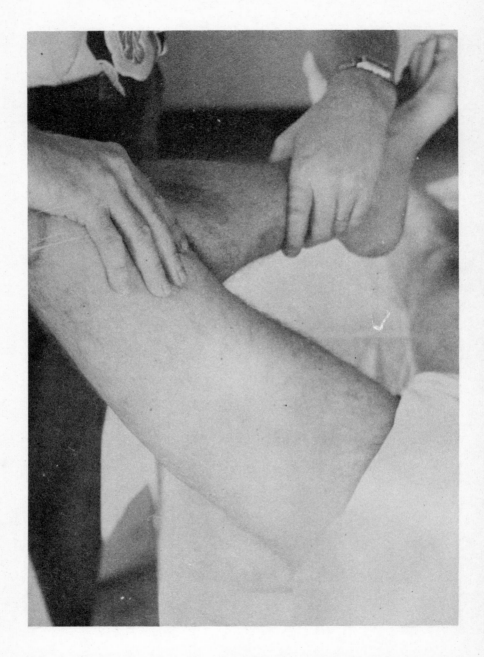

FLEXION FOLLOWED BY EXTENSION AND ABDUCTION WILL
STRETCH THE MUSCLES AND INCREASE PAIN ON MOTION.

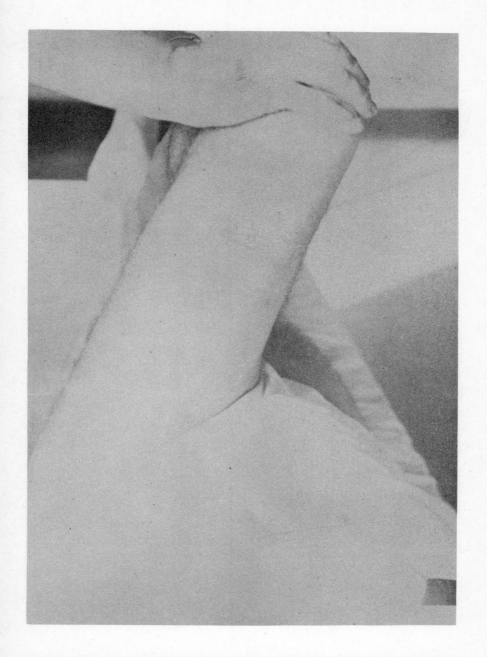

FLEXION OF THIGH ON PELVIS AND PELVIS ON ABDOMEN
RELAXES THESE MUSCLES AND MINIMIZES PAIN. OTHER
MOTIONS NOT PAINFUL IN PSOASITIS.

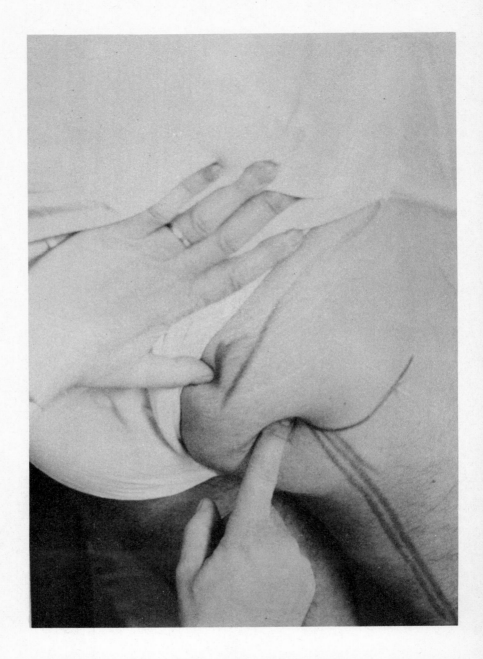

POSTERIOR MYOSITIS INVOLVING THE EXTERNAL ROTATORS OF THE THIGH PRODUCES PAIN AT POSTERIOR ASPECT OF HIP JOINT, PAIN ON PRESSURE OVER AREA.

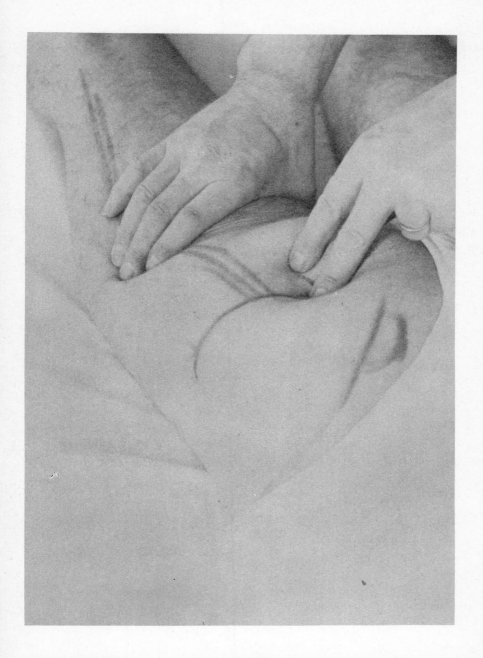

PAIN OVER SCIATIC NERVE, SUPERIOR AND INFERIOR GE-
MELLI, QUADRATUS FEMORIS, PYRIFORMIS, BICEPS FEMORIS.

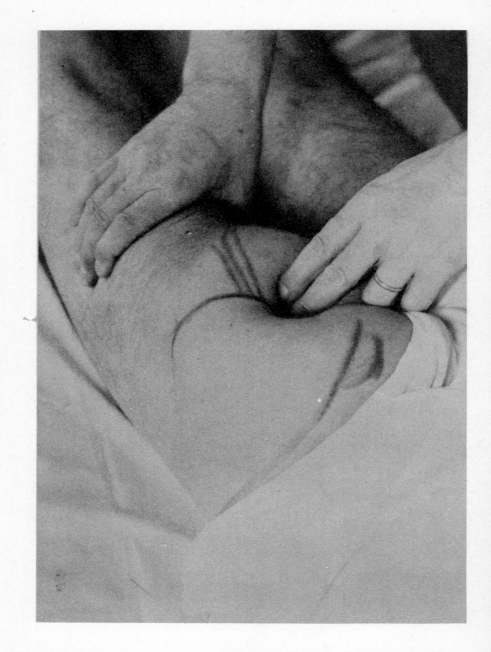

PRESSURE ON SCIATIC NERVE MAY GIVE TRAJECTORY STAB
OF PAIN.

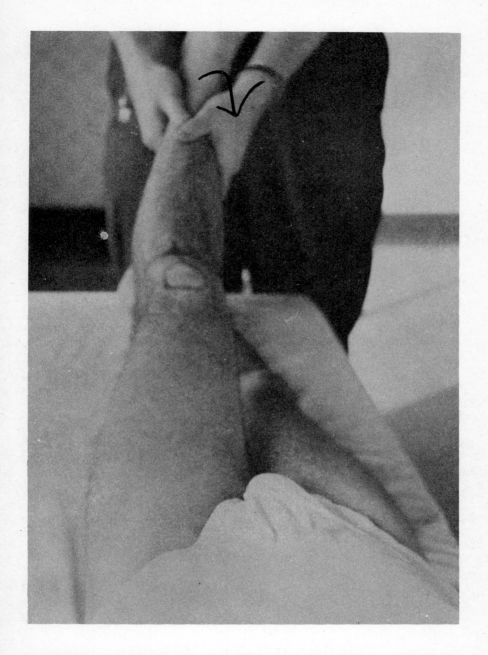

INTERNAL ROTATION OF LEG AND THIGH PUTS A STRETCH ON THE EXTERNAL ROTATORS AND INCREASES PAIN. EXTERNAL ROTATION RELAXES THOSE MUSCLES AND RELIEVES POSTERIOR MYOSITIC PAIN.

MEDIAL HIP AREA

Adductor myositis is the usual source of pain in this area. It may seem local but will be found hyperesthetic down the insertion of the muscle.

Adductor myositis is usually due to weight shift from the side of involvement but may be due to other causes, reflex or traumatic.

Acquisition of symmetrical weight bearing should precede local treatment. Local treatment is the treatment of myositis as outlined before.

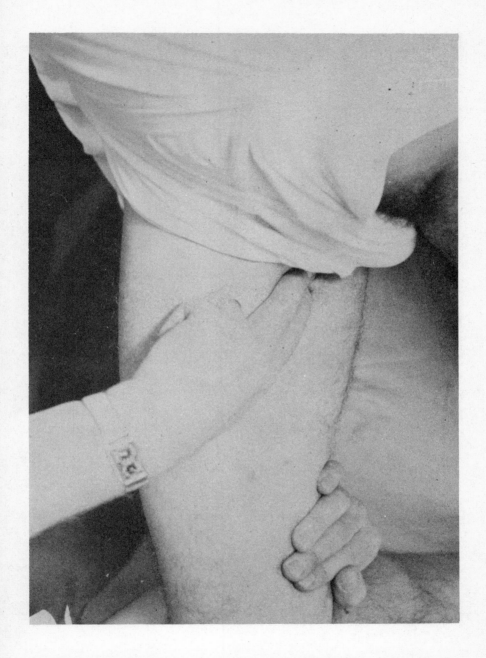

ADDUCTOR MYOSITIS. USUALLY ON SIDE OF ACTUAL OR
RELATIVE SHORT . EXTREMITY. PAIN ALONG COURSE OF
ADDUCTOR MUSCLES, MORE MARKED IN BILATERAL WEIGHT
BEARING.

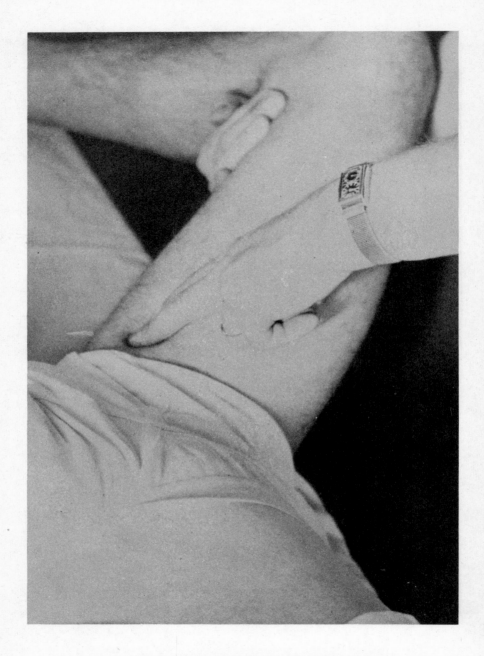

FURTHER ABDUCTION INCREASES PAIN.

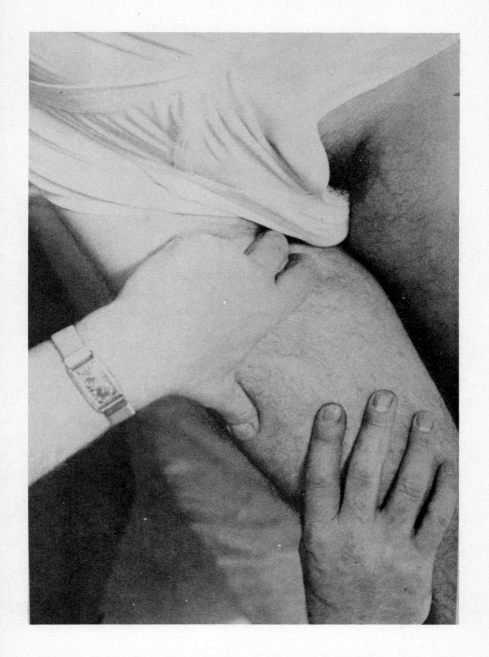

ADDUCTION RELAXES MUSCLE AND DIMINISHES PAIN. NO OTHER MOTIONS ARE PAINFUL IN ADDUCTOR MYOSITIS.

LATERAL HIP AREA

Pain may be pointed at the greater trochanter but usually will extend also from the outer lip of the crest of the ilium to the fibular head and lateral knee joint capsule.

The usual factor causing the tensor fascia lata myositis and iliotibial band fascitis is weight shift toward the affected side, which places much stress on the lateral guy. Fascitis, of course, may be primary, reflex, and/or due to trauma.

Treatment: removal of the tiological factor and stretching of the band and muscle. Local treatment as in any myositis will be effective.

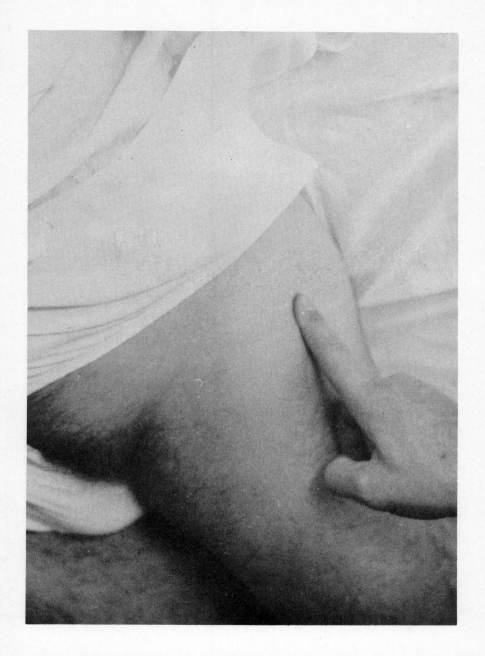

PAIN OVER GREATER TROCHANTER SIMULATED BY ILIO-
TIBIAL BAND AND TENSOR FASCIA LATA TENSION. USUALLY
ON ACTUAL OR RELATIVE LONG LEG SIDE, INCREASED BY
FULL WEIGHT BEARING ON THAT LEG. PATIENT CONSCIOUS
OF SPOT PAIN OVER BONE PROMINENCE.

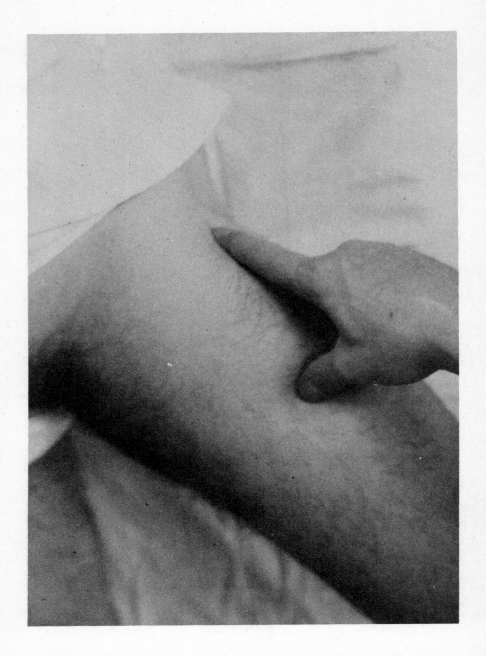

HYPERESTHESIA AND PAIN WILL BE FOUND ALL ALONG THE COURSE FROM THE CREST OF THE ILIUM TO THE LATERAL TIBIAL ATTACHMENT. FURTHER ABDUCTION DIMINISHES PAIN.

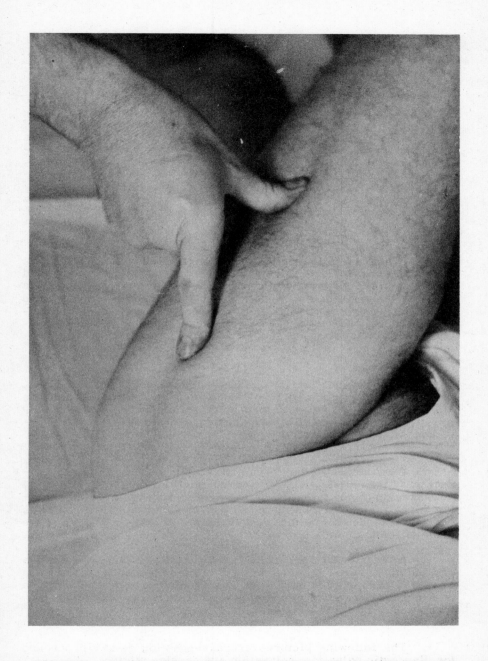

FORCED ADDUCTION INCREASES PAIN. NO OTHER HIP MO-
TIONS PAINFUL.

GENERAL CONSIDERATIONS OF SPINAL AREA

Palpation and passive motion have a dual purpose in the spinal area. First, while placing an area thru motion, palpation of spinous, transverse, or articular processes will reveal perversion of motion. Secondly, passive motion has the favorable effect of relaxing musculature and facilitating venous and lymphatic return.

Diagnosis of the area, type of lesion, and the relative amounts of fibrosis and/or hypertonicity is essential before motion correction can be properly applied.

After such is determined, then thorough relaxation of muscle hypertonicity should be obtained. Such relaxation is usually and easily obtained by mild inhibitive pressure, mild stretching of the belly or the ends of the muscle group. It is important that this manipulative process be slow and deliberate. Any sudden application of force, too much force, or a sudden release, results in mechanical stimulation to the muscle and an increase in the hypertonicity.

When manual relaxation fails, one may resort to diathermy, packs, motion equipment, tape, analgesics and sedatives, calcium gluconate 10cc 10% sol. I.V., procaine infiltration, nerve blocks, or intravenous procaine. Tolserol and tubo-crurare and other substances may be of value.

When relaxation has been accomplished, specific lesion correction is then attempted. Fibrous restrictions and adhesions must be broken down and the average range of motion acquired by carrying the articulations thru their full range of motion. Obviously this corrective force will be the least traumatic if it is in the line of the plane of the articulation.

After motion correction is accomplished, the articulations are put thru their complete range of motion frequently. This is an essential part of treatment that is all too often neglected. Motion is necessary to return circulation, and essential to prevent the reformation of multiple adhesions.

The following pictures are a suggestion as to a procedure for diagnostic palpation, relaxation and passive motion.

PALPATION FOR SEGMENTAL

MOTION

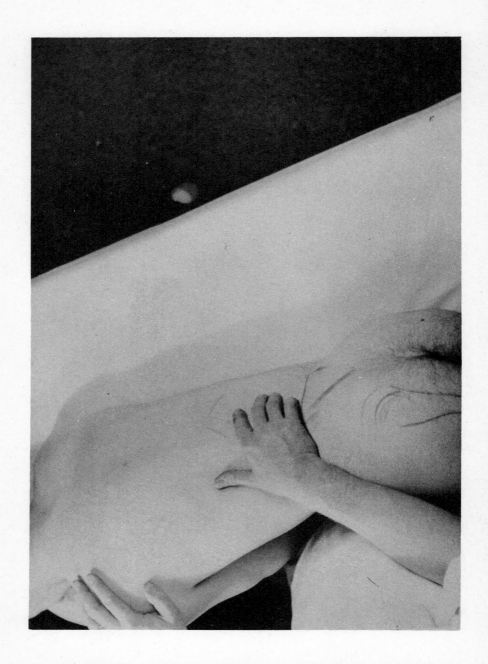

PALPATION OR PASSIVE MOTION ACQUIRED WITH THORACIC
LEVERAGE. MOSTLY APPLICABLE TO THORACIC AREA.

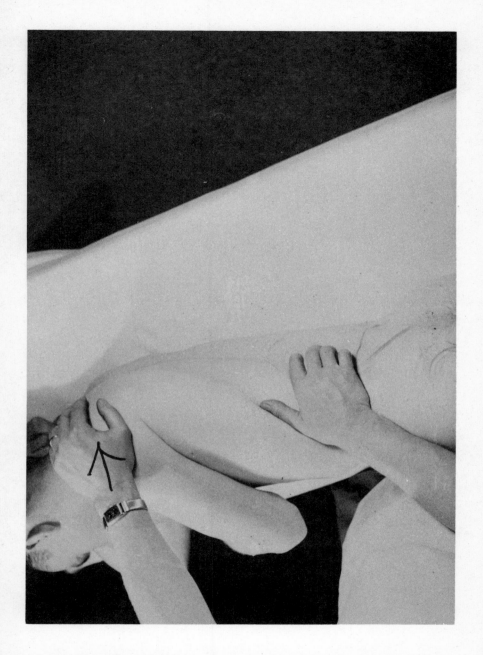

CEPHALIC HAND ROLLS LATERALLY AND PATIENT'S SHOUL-
DER PRODUCES LATERAL FLEXION WITH ROTATION. SPIN-
OUS PROCESS MOTION IS PALPATED.

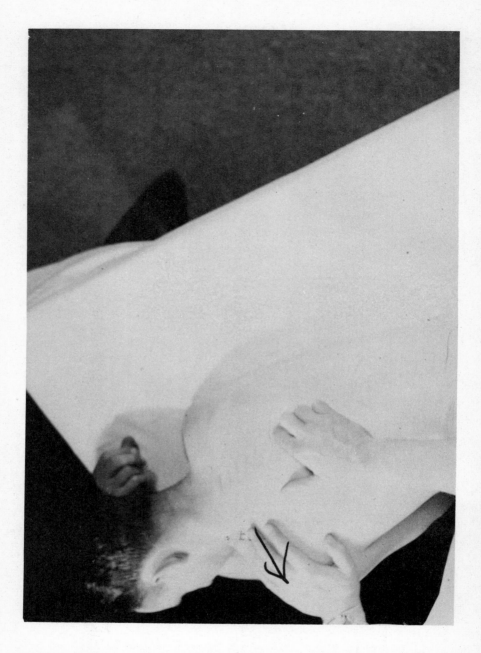

SHOULDER IS PULLED FORWARD, PRODUCING LATERAL
FLEXION WITH ROTATION TO OPPOSITE SIDE. SUCH SEG-
MENTALLY CONTRIBUTIVE MOTION SHOULD BE PRESENT
AND PALPABLE.

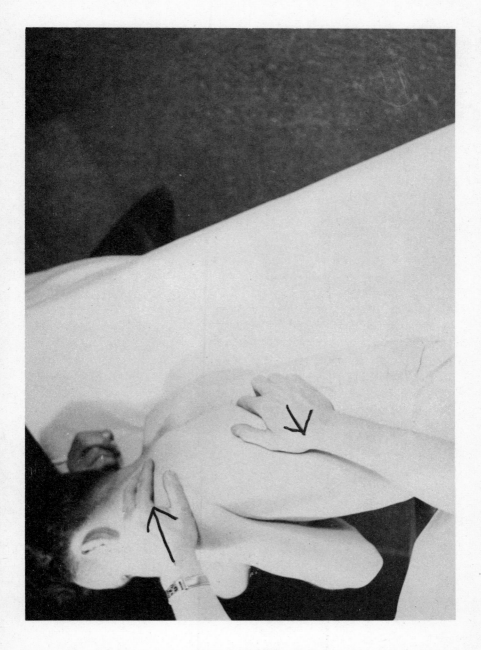

MUSCLE RELAXATION MAY BE ACQUIRED BY SAME MOTIONS.

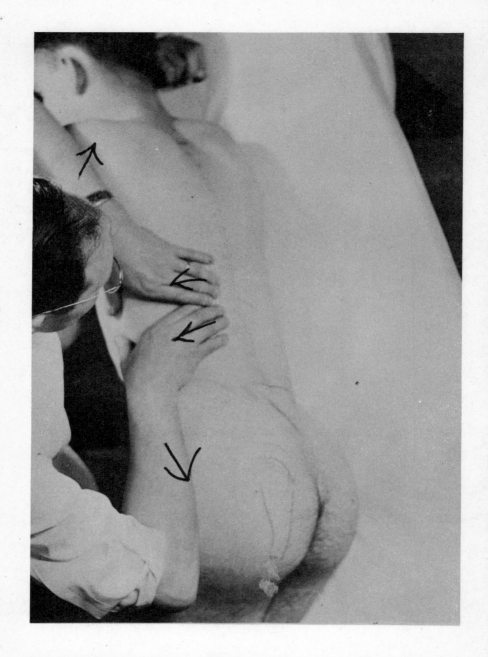

SEPARATION OF SHOULDER AND PELVIS WHILE EXTENDING
THE INTERVENING SPINE. THIS IS APPLICABLE IN PREG-
NANCY AND AT THE BEDSIDE FOR EASY PASSIVE MOTION
AND MOTION FOR LESION DIAGNOSIS.

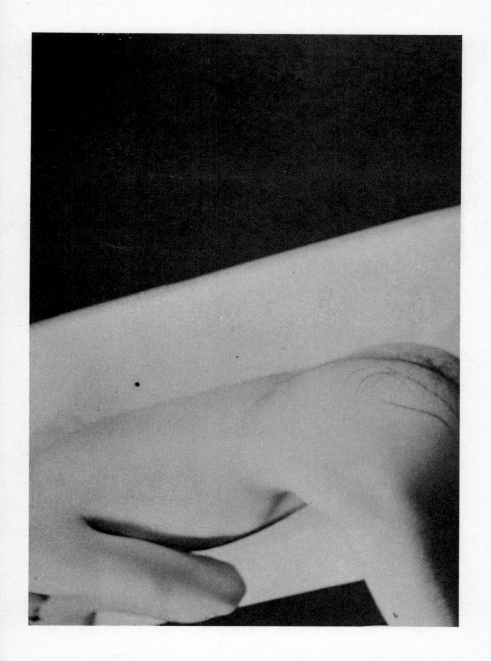

MOTION PALPATION - PATIENT ON SIDE WITH LEGS AND THIGHS FLEXED AND EXTENDING BEYOND SIDE OF TABLE.

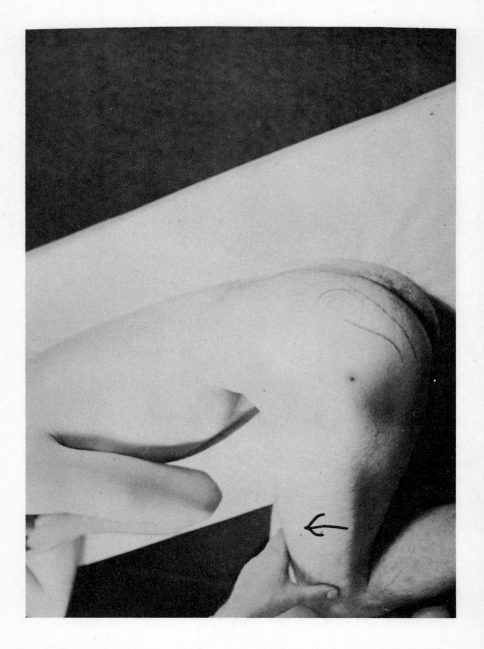

PATIENT'S KNEES ARE CAUGHT WITH CAUDAL HAND AND
PHYSICIAN'S THIGH SO THE PELVIS CAN BE FLEXED AND
EXTENDED EASILY.

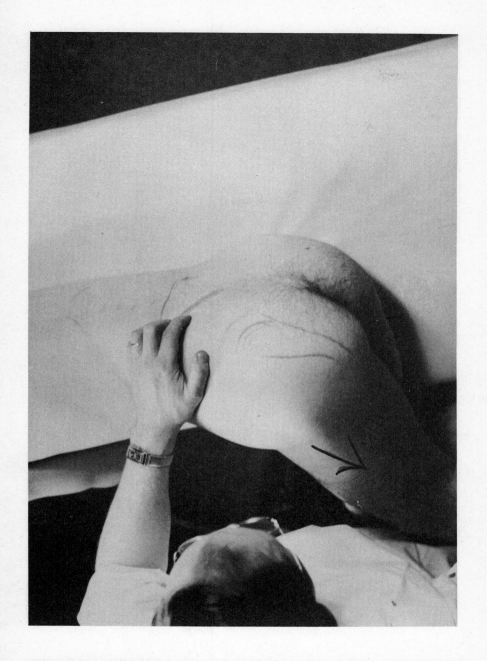

PALPATING SACRO-ILIAC MOTION WITH THIGH AND ILIUM FLEXED AND EXTENDED.

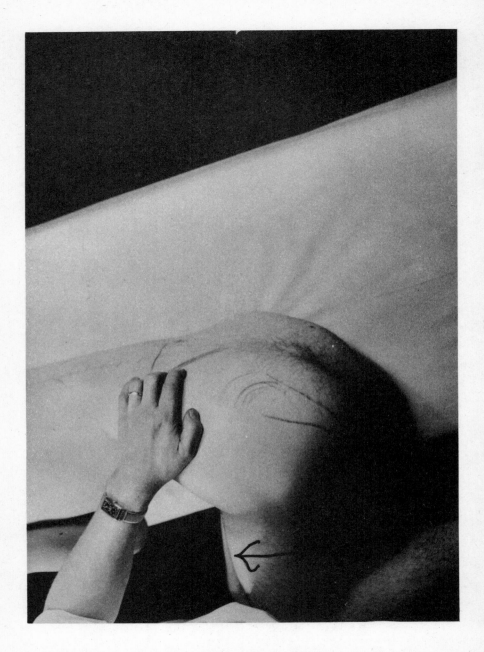

ILIUM SHOULD ROCK BACKWARD, DEEPENING SACRAL GROOVE,
WHEN THIGH AND PELVIS ARE FLEXED.

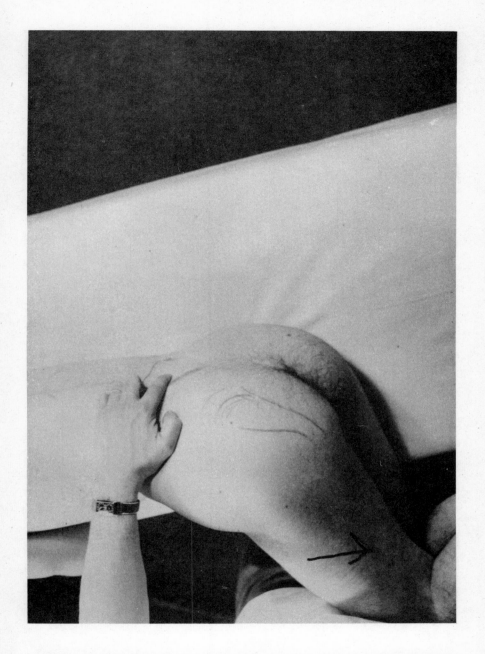

ILIUM SHOULD MOVE FORWARD, EXTENDING SACRUM WHEN
THIGH AND PELVIS ARE EXTENDED.

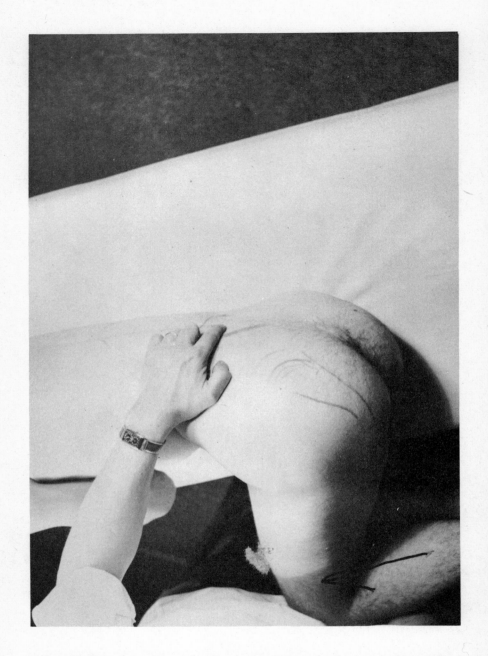

FLEXION OF BOTH THIGHS AND PELVIS SHOULD FLEX LUM-
BOSACRAL ARTICULATIONS AND SEPARATE SPINOUS PROC-
ESSES IF MOTION IS NOT RESTRICTED.

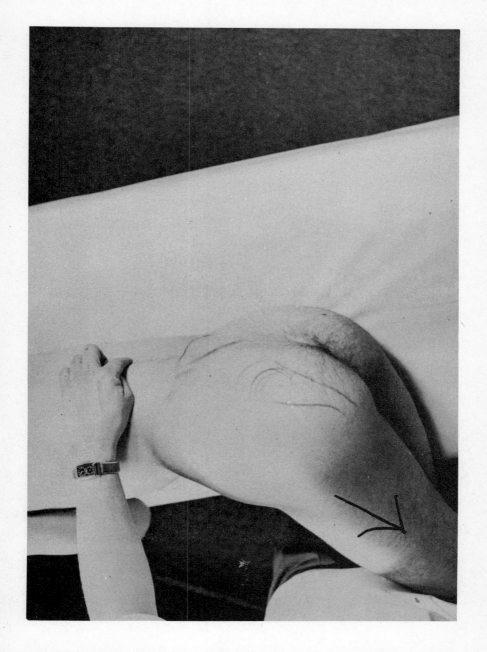

EXTENSION OF THIGHS AND PELVIS SHOULD, IF MOTION IS
PRESENT, APPROXIMATE SPINOUS PROCESSES.

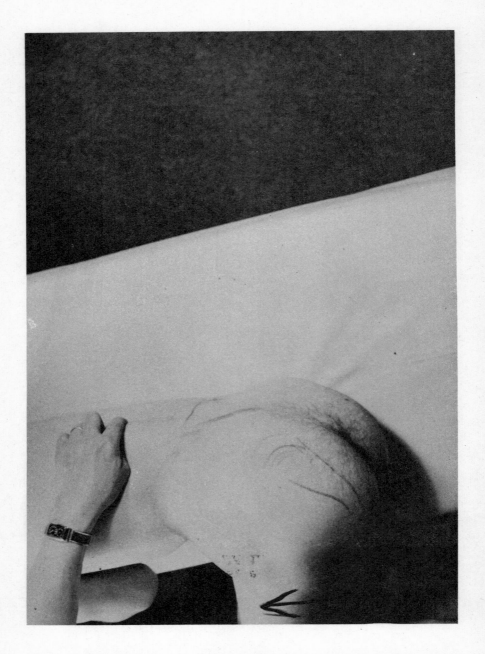

THIS TEST MAY BE USED THRU SACRO-ILIAC, LUMBAR AND
MOST OF THE THORACIC AREA.

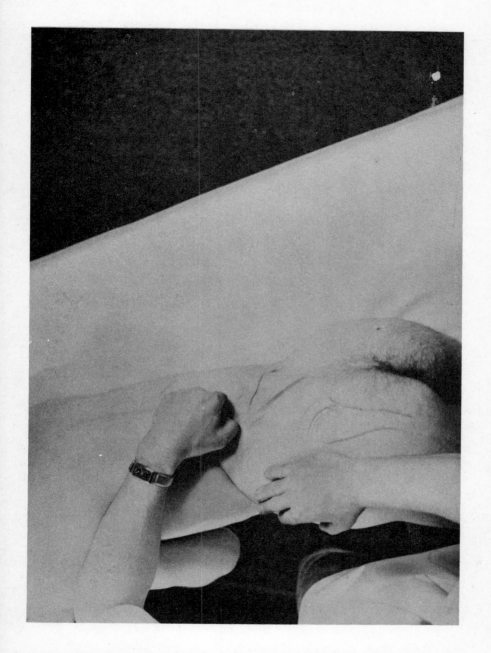

AN ALTERNATIVE TECHNIQUE FOR PALPATION OF MOTION,
WITH ONE HAND PALPATING THE SPINOUS PROCESSES.

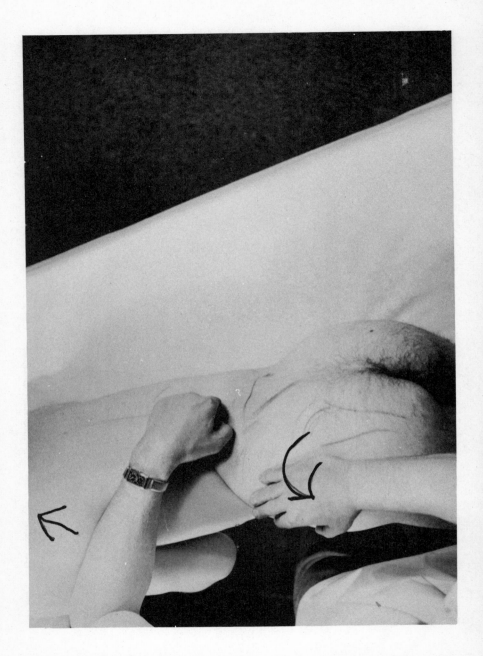

THE OTHER HAND ROCKS THE ILIUM FORWARD AND BACK-
WARD. PATIENT ANCHORED ON TABLE WITH THE ARM OF
THE PALPATING HAND.

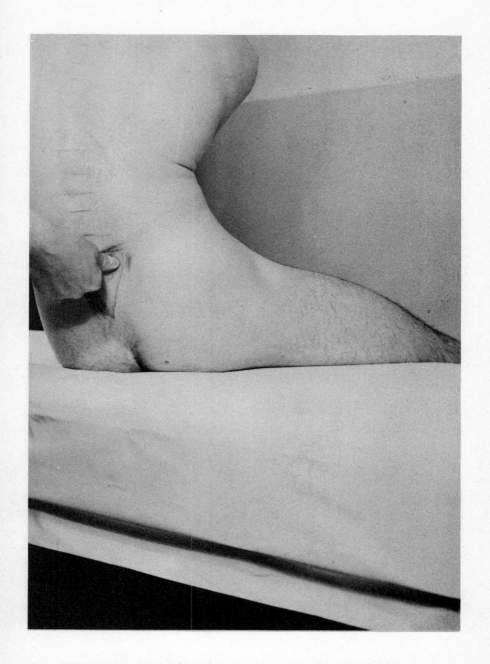

SAME PALPATION EVIDENCE MAY BE ELICITED WITH PA-
TIENT SITTING, PUTTING ENTIRE SPINAL AREA THRU FLEX-
ION, EXTENSION, LATERAL FLEXION WITH ROTATION; WITH
OTHER HAND DETECTING MOTION AT SACRO-ILIAC OR THE
INTERSPINOUS OR RIB AREAS.

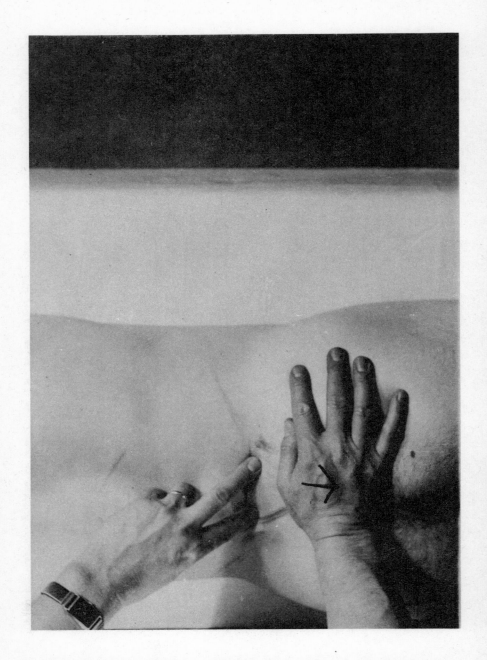

SACRO-ILIAC MOBILITY MAY BE PALPATED AT THOSE AR-
TICULATIONS, WHILE THE OTHER HAND OVER THE CONVEX-
ITY OF THE SACRUM ROCKS IT BACKWARD INTO EXTEN-
SION.

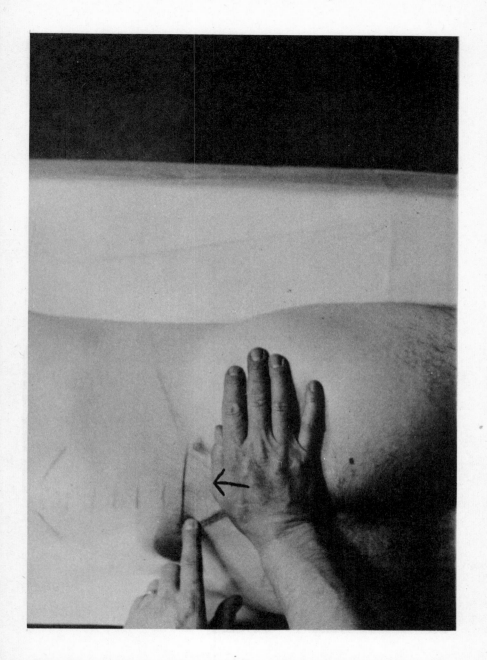

MOVING CAUDAL HAND UPWARD, THE PRESSURE WILL FLEX
THE TOP OF SACRUM. MOTION PALPATED AT SACRO-ILIAC
ARTICULATION.

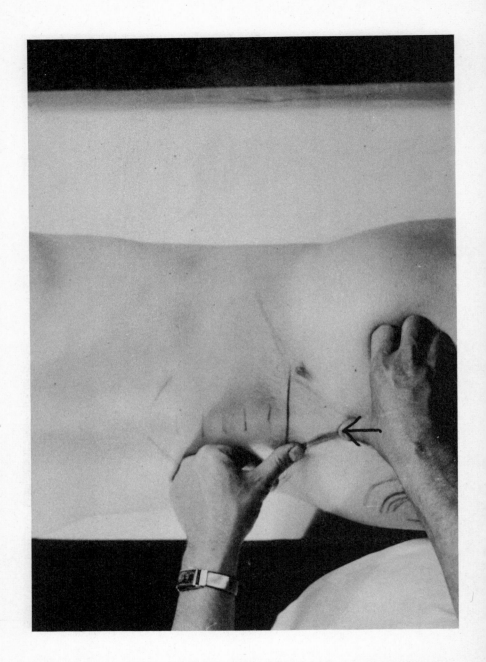

UNILATERAL MOTION MAY BE PALPATED ALTERNATELY WITH ONE THUMB, THEN THE OTHER. FORCE DIVERGES LATERALLY 45° WITH PLANE OF ARTICULATION. LOWER THUMB FORCES SACRUM INTO EXTENSION.

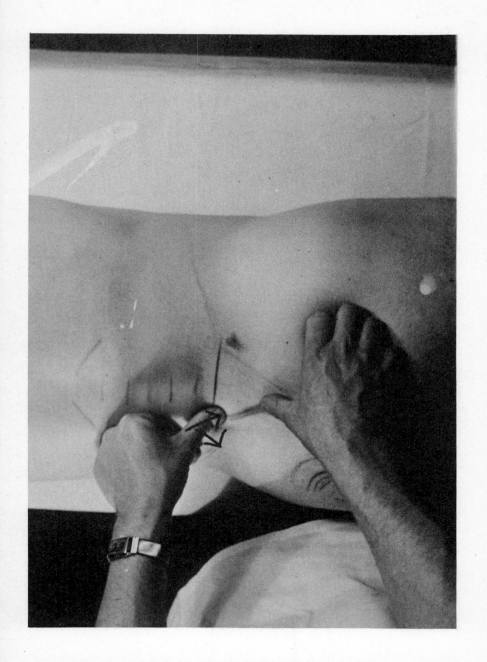

UPPER THUMB FORCES SACRUM INTO FLEXION. MOTION
PALPATED BY RESTING THUMB.

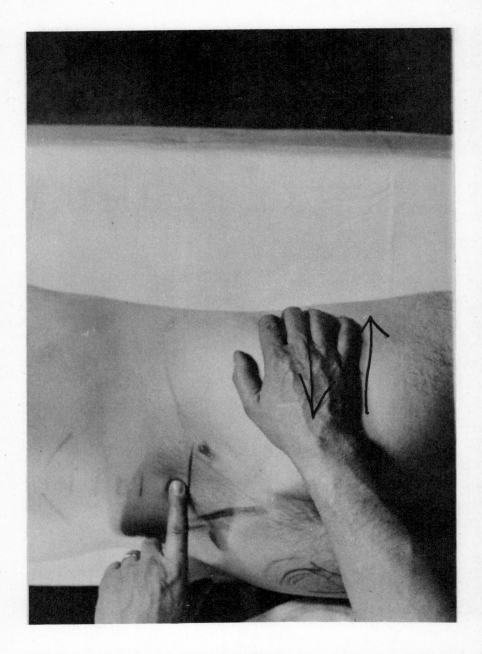

PALPATION OF SPINOUS PROCESS MOTION WHILE CAUDAL
HAND ROLLS PELVIS, PRODUCING LATERAL FLEXION AND
ROTATION.

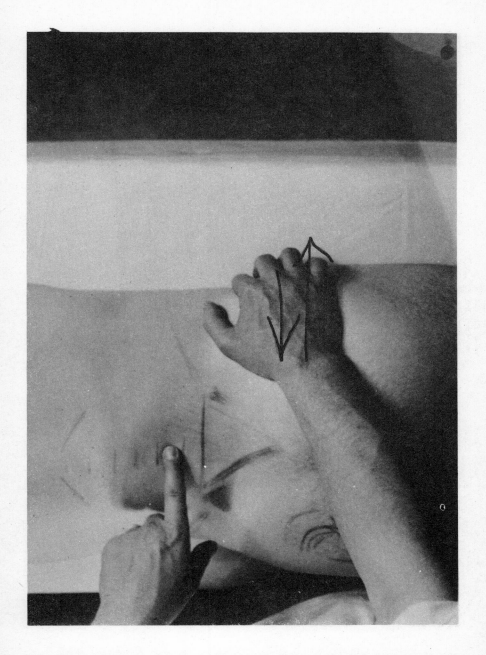

ROCKING PELVIS WHILE PALPATING SPINOUS PROCESSES.

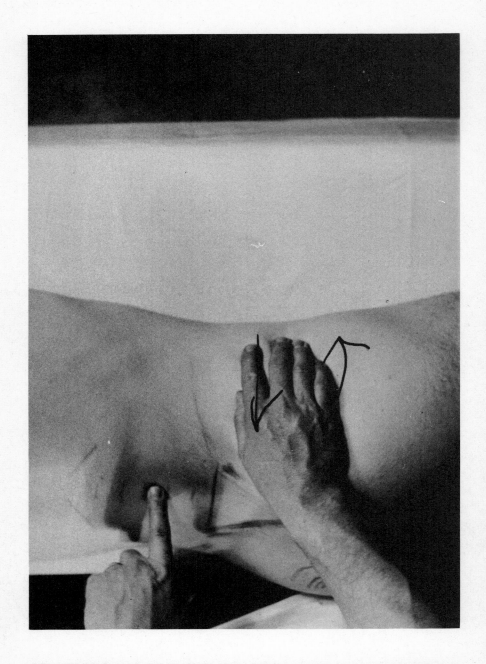

ROCKING PELVIS WHILE PALPATING SPINOUS PROCESSES.
THIS MAY BE CARRIED UPWARD TO THE MID THORACIC
AREA OR HIGHER.

MUSCLE RELAXATION AND PASSIVE

MOTION

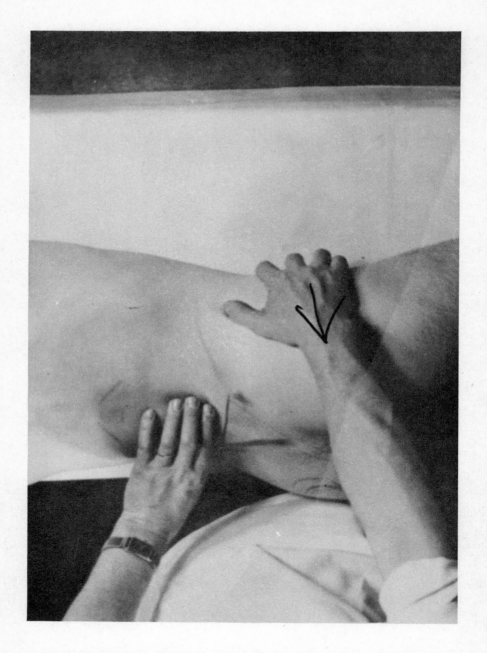

PALPATION FOR MOTION TO LOCALIZE AREAS OF HYPER-
TONICITY OF MUSCLE AND IMPAIRED MOBILITY SHOULD BE
CARRIED UPWARD SEGMENT BY SEGMENT. PALPATION BE-
TWEEN SPINOUS PROCESSES WHILE THE AREA IS MOBILIZED
WITH THE OTHER HAND.

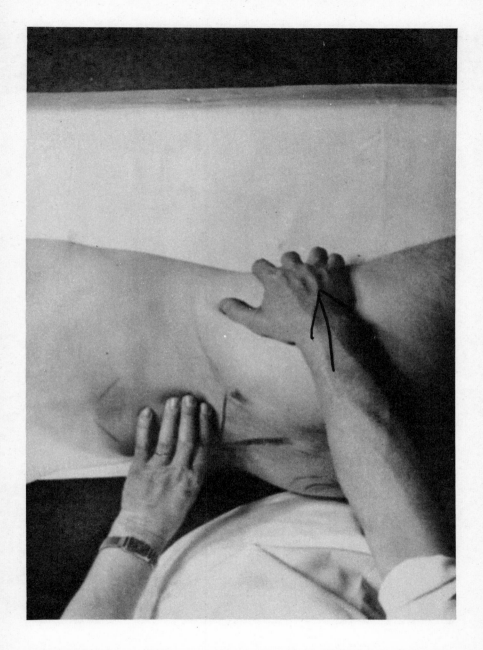

PALPATION OF SEGMENTAL MUSCULATURE AND MOTION
RELATIONS AT THE TRANSVERSE PROCESS AREA, ALONG
WITH SKIN AND MUSCLE TEXTURE AND TEMPERATURE, USU-
ALLY IS PALPABLY NOTICEABLE OF SEGMENTAL DISTURB-
ANCES.

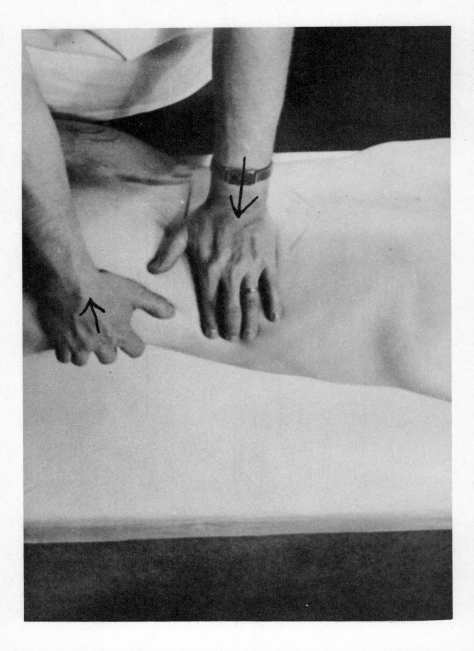

STRETCHING OF MUSCLE TO DETECT REBOUND HYPERTON-
ICITY OR RELAXATION IS A VALUABLE DIAGNOSTIC FINDING.

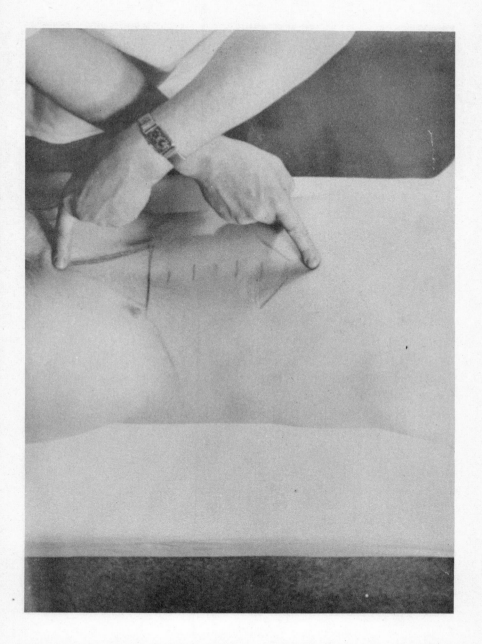

REDUCTION OF LUMBO-SACRAL ANGULATION AND LUMBAR
INDEX IS EFFECTIVE GENERAL RELAXATION TREATMENT
AND ALSO STRETCHES THE LUMBAR MUSCULATURE.

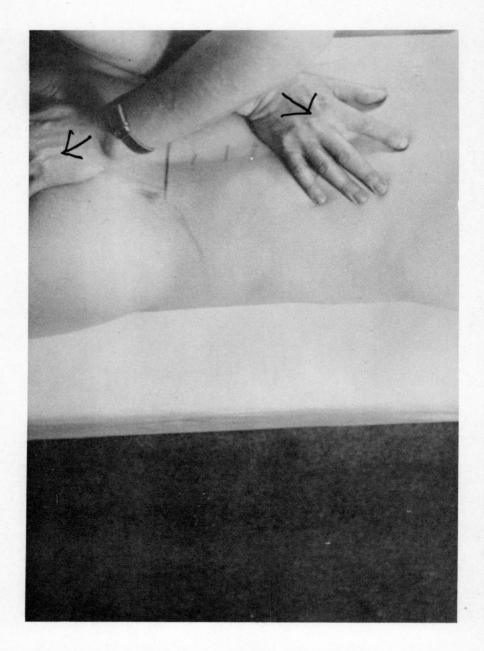

CROSSING THE ARMS AND THEN MERELY DROPPING STATIC
WEIGHT ON ARMS AND HANDS WILL STRETCH THE LUMBAR
SPINE AND REDUCE ITS EXTENDED POSITION.

134

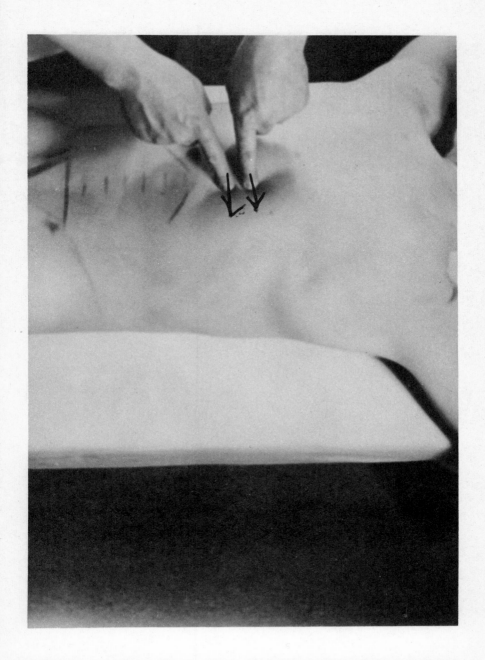

MUSCULATURE IS RELAXED BY STRETCHING THE ENDS OF
THE MUSCLE OR BY STRETCHING THE BELLY. HENCE THE
PARAVERTEBRAL MUSCULATURE IS PUSHED AWAY FROM
THE SPINOUS PROCESS AREA, SLOWLY AND EVENLY.

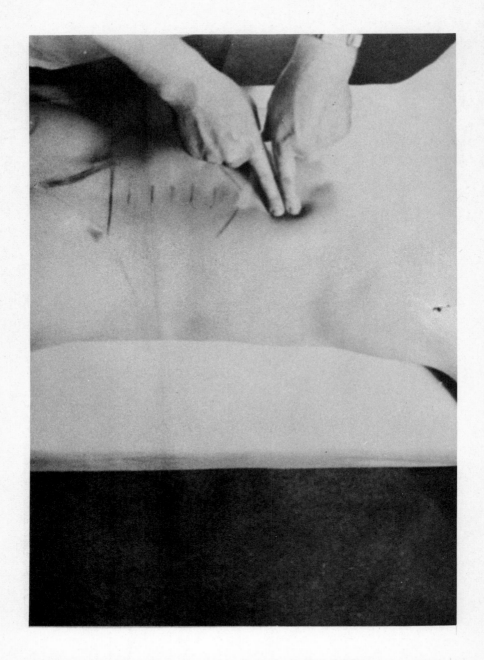

MUSCULATURE IS RELAXED BY FIRM DEEP PRESSURE. HENCE PRESSURE AT RIGHT ANGLES TO THE LONG AXIS OF THE MUSCLE AIDS RELAXATION IF ADMINISTERED SLOWLY AND EVENLY.

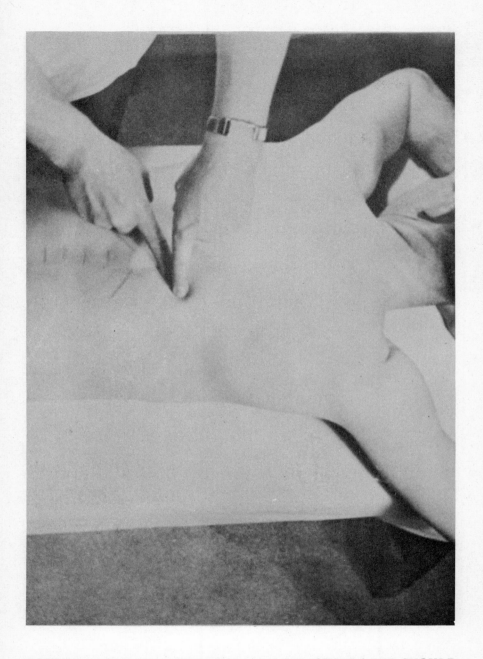

FORCES ABOVE AND SUBSEQUENTLY DEMONSTRATED SHOULD ALSO BE CARRIED LATERALLY BETWEEN THE RIBS FOR EFFECT ON THE INTERCOSTALS.

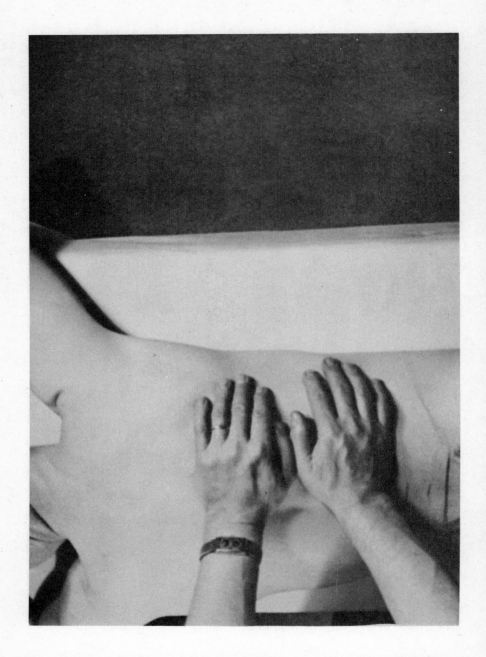

PATIENTS FACE TOWARD PHYSICIAN - PHYSICIAN'S HANDS
BEYOND SPINOUS PROCESSES - THUS AVOIDING EXTENSOR
REFLEX ON SIDE TOWARD WHICH CHIN IS TURNED.

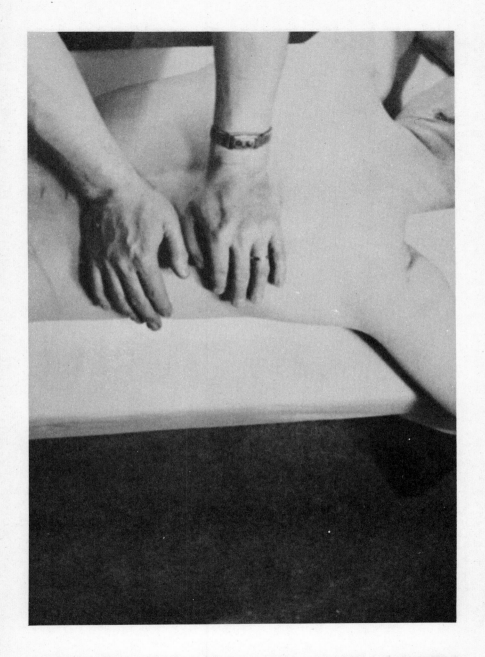

WEIGHT IS SWUNG SLOWLY AND EVENLY ONTO STRAIGHTENED
ARMS AND HANDS PUSHING MUSCLE LATERALLY.

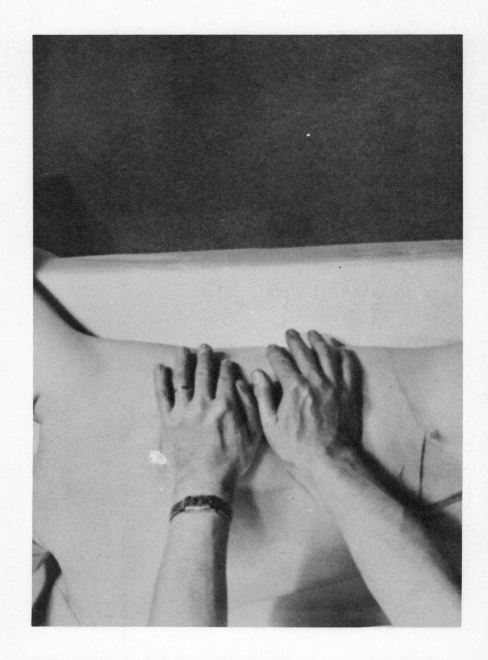

WITH 25 TO 50 LBS. APPLIED, IT IS HELD FOR SEVERAL
SECONDS. THEN EQUALLY AS SLOWLY AND EVENLY THE
WEIGHT AND INHIBITORY PRESSURE IS GRADUALLY REMOVED.

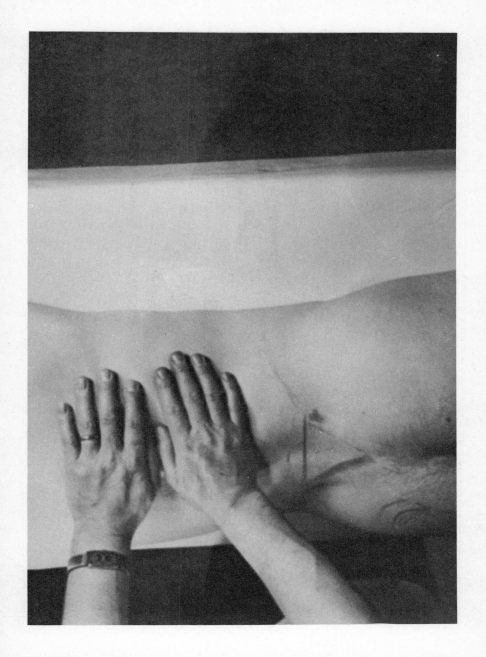

ONE OR TWO SUCH APPLICATIONS IS USUALLY ADEQUATE.

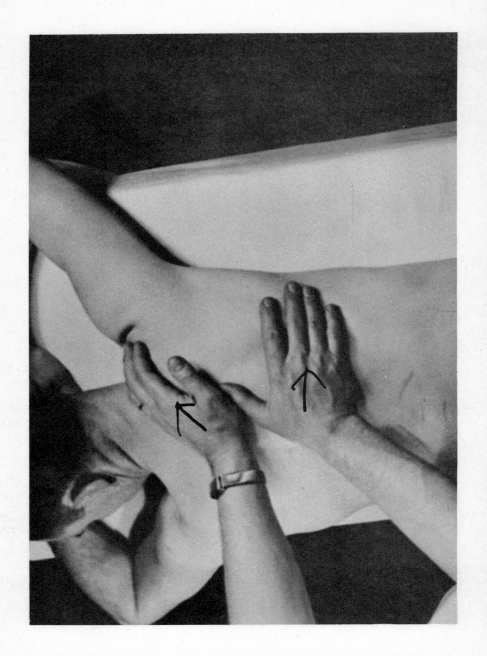

SAME SLOW EVEN FORCES CARRIED UPWARD TO THE CIR-
CUMSCAPULAR MUSCLES.

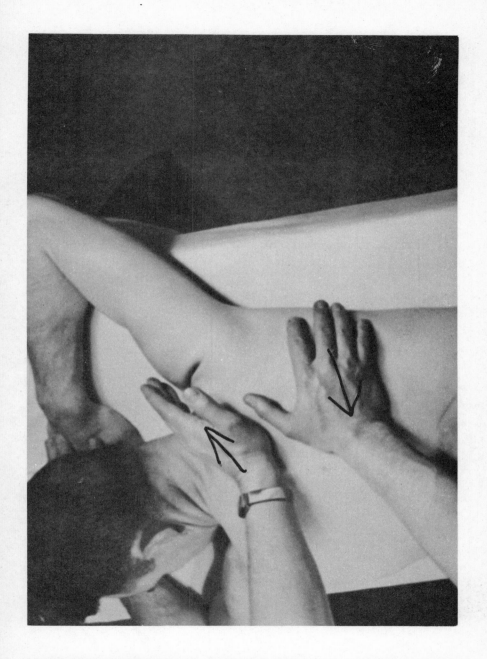

SAME MILD STRETCHING CARRIED EVENLY UP TO LEVATOR
ANGULAE SCAPULAE, RHOMBOIDEI AND UPPER BORDERS OF
TRAPEZIUS.

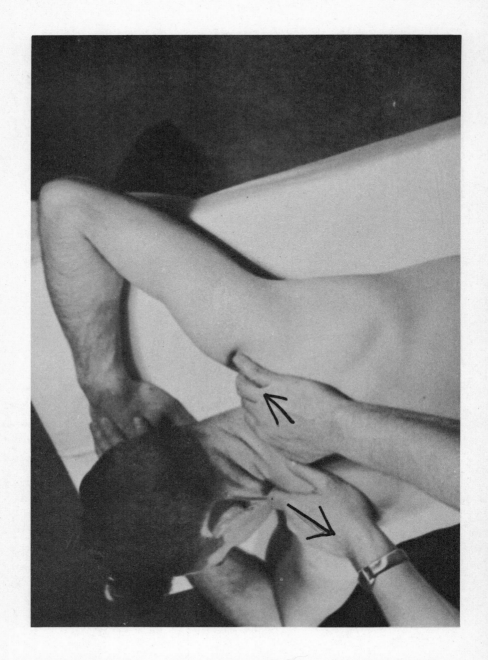

PULLING MILDLY ON THESE MUSCLES AT RIGHT ANGLES
TO THEIR LONG AXIS ON ONE SIDE, WHILE PUSHING IN THE
DIRECTION OF THEIR LONG AXIS ON THE OTHER, GIVES
MOTION AND RELAXATION.

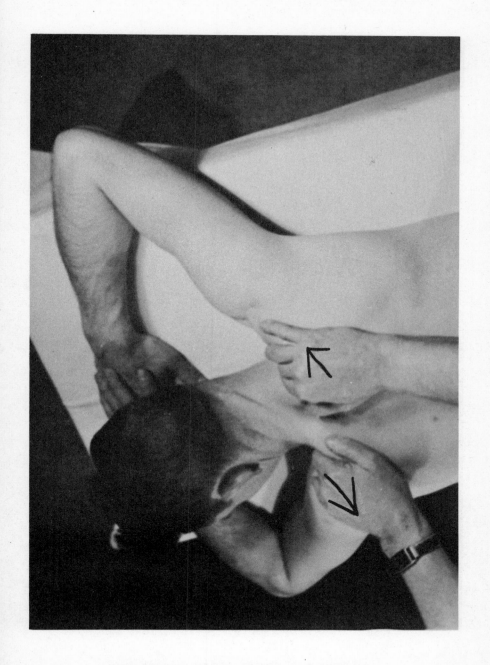

SAME AS ABOVE - SLOW AND EASY

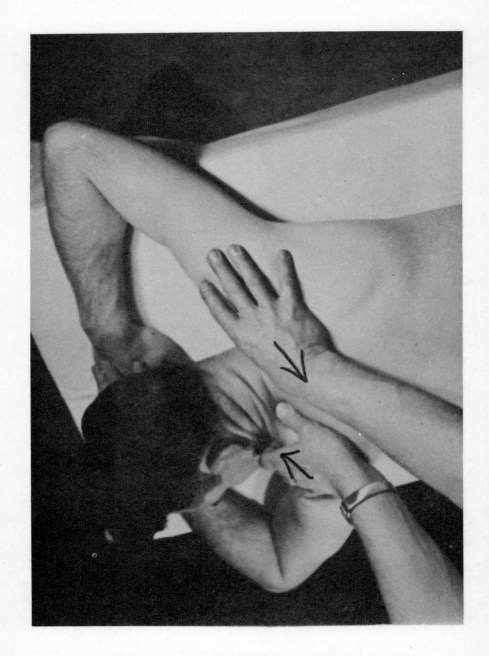

REVERSAL OF DIRECTION OF FORCE

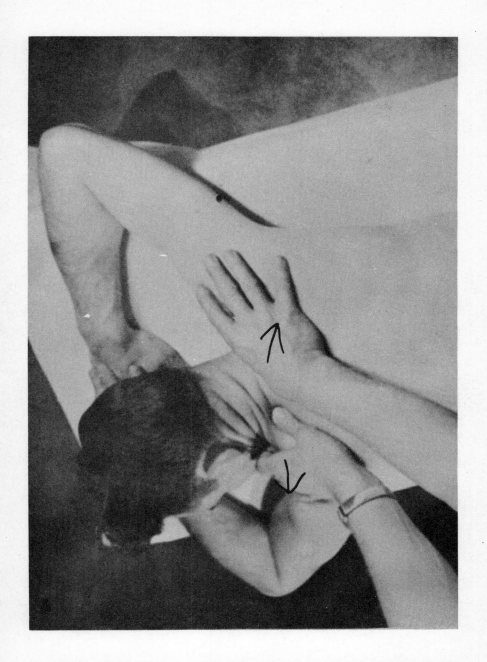

BILATERALLY EQUAL FORCES SHOULD BE USED AND MAY
BE SYNCHRONOUSLY IN THE SAME OR ANTAGONISTIC DI-
RECTIONS. IMPORTANT THAT SUCH MANIPULATIONS BE
SLOWLY, EVENLY, AND FIRMLY APPLIED WITH A SLOW
GRADUAL RELEASE.

SACRO-ILIAC ARTICULATION

SACRO-ILIAC ARTICULATIONS

This articulation is a bi-limbed articulation. The short vertical limb has its plane of motion directed from postero-superior or extended base position to antero-inferiorly or flexion base position. In this motion bilateral flexion or extension the motion at the long or horizontal limb is across the articulation. The axis of flexion extension motion is thru the posterior portion of the body of the second sacral segment or, by other authority, the tubercle on the back of the second sacral segment. Outline of the physical findings of these types of lesions will be found below.

We, for practical purposes, visualize the axis of rotation in torsion to run longitudinally thru the body of the sacrum, even tho it actually shifts slightly toward the posterior or extended sacral side at the sacral base and toward the flexed sacral side caudally. In torsion there is a twist around the long axis and a tilt to the sacral top downward toward the flexed sacral side. Physical findings in torsion charted below.

Sacral descent occurs due to trauma in which the sacrum usually descends vertically, driven deeper between the ilia without movement along physiological planes of motion mentioned. The roughened irregular articular surfaces of the articulations may be impinged by sacral descent sufficiently that motion is nullified-- even corrective motion applied to a flexed, extended, or torsioned sacrum locked in one of those positions by sacral descent.

Diagnosis of sacral descent must be made from the history. Treatment must be straight leg traction in the anatomical position. Sacral ascent may be acquired and produce a transitory hypermobility. Gravity however, usually will settle the sacrum to normal position as far as its horizontal anatomical position.

	BILATERAL FLEXION OF SACRUM	BILATERAL EXTENSION OF SACRUM
Top of sacrum	Antero-inferior	Postero-superior
Last sacral segment	Postero-superior	Antero-inferior
Sacro-tuberous and Sacro-spinous ligament	Tight	Lax
Posterior Superior Iliac Spine	Prominent	Less prominent
Sacral Groove	Deep	Shallow
Lumbo-sacral angle	Increased	Decreased
Lumbar Index	Increased	Decreased
Anterior Superior Iliac Spine- acetabulum	Relatively elevated	Relatively lowered

150

SACRAL TORSION

Slight differences exist between typical flexion findings on the one side and extension findings on the other. These are produced by the rotation of the whole sacrum roughly around its longitudinal axis. Hence on the flexed side or the side from which the body of sacrum rotates, the whole side of the sacrum moves anterior and inferiorly; whereas on the extended side, that half of the sacrum moves postero-superiorly.

SACRAL TORSION

	FLEXION SIDE	EXTENSION SIDE
Whole side of sacrum	Antero-inferior	Postero-superior
Sacral groove	Deep	Shallow
Post. Sup. Iliac Spine	Prominent and caudad	Less prominent and cephalic
Sacral top	Low	Elevated
Sacro-tuberous and Sacro-spinous lig.	Relaxed	Tight
Last sacral segment	Less prominent	More prominent and shifted toward this side.
Anterior Sup. Iliac Spine and acetabulum	Relatively elevated	Relatively lowered

Compensatory curve often present in lumbar spine, convex to flexed sacral side.

Extended lumbo-sacral facet usually present on extended sacral side.

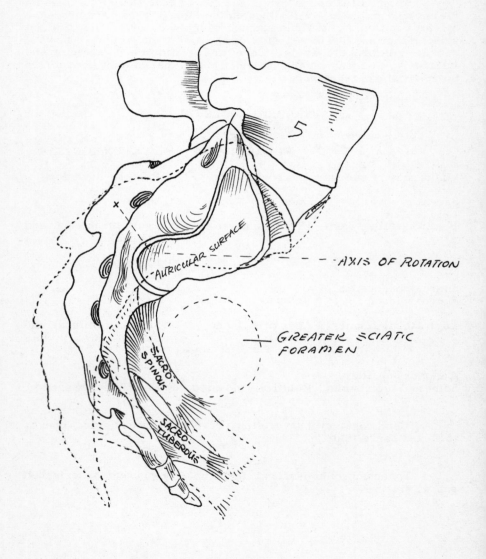

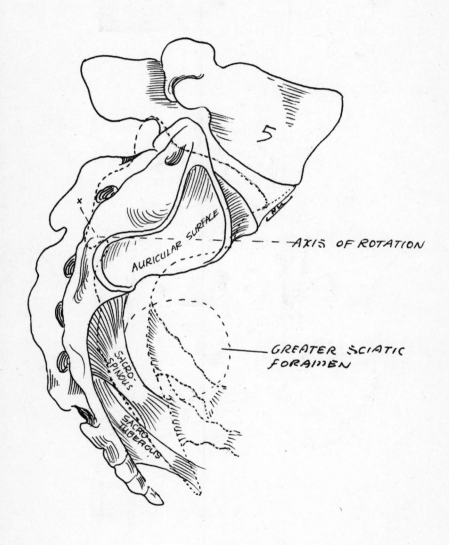

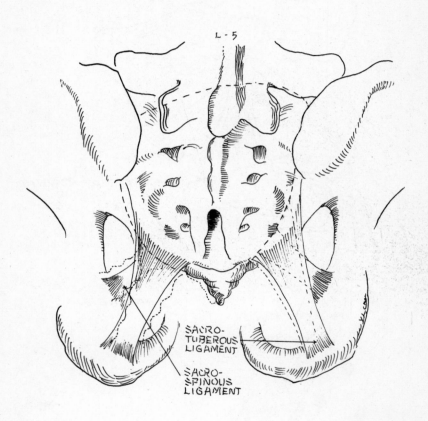

L - 5

SACRO-
TUBEROUS
LIGAMENT

SACRO-
SPINOUS
LIGAMENT

FLEXED SACRUM
LATERAL TECHNIC

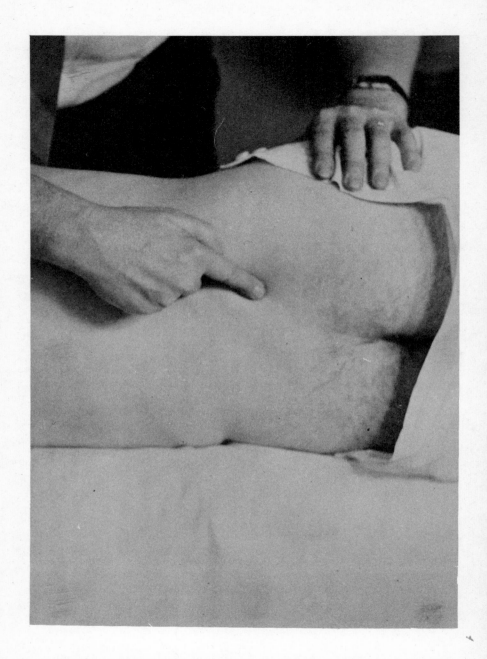

LATERAL TECHNIQUE USUAL FOR BOTH SIDES OF A BI-
LATERAL SACRAL FLEXION OR FOR THE FLEXED SIDE OF
A SACRAL TORSION. PALPATING THE DEEP SACRAL GROOVE
AND PROMINENT CAUDAL POSTERIOR SUPERIOR ILIAC SPINE.

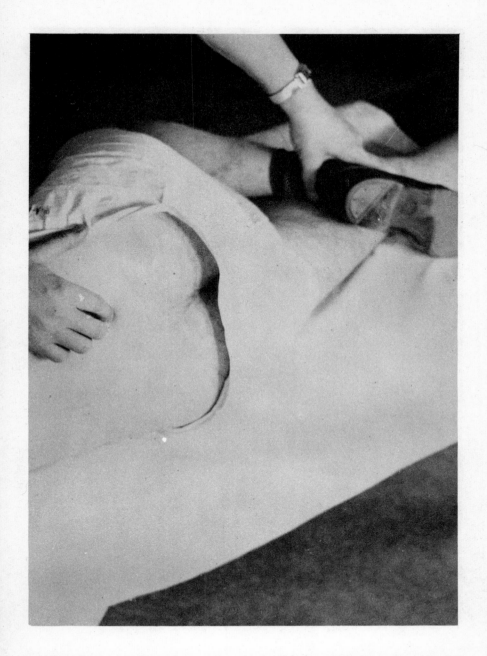

LOWER LEG STRAIGHT. UPPER LEG FLEXED WITH FOOT
LOCKED IN POPLITEAL SPACE TO PREVENT LEG FALLING
OFF TABLE TO BECOME AN ANTAGONISTIC WEIGHT.

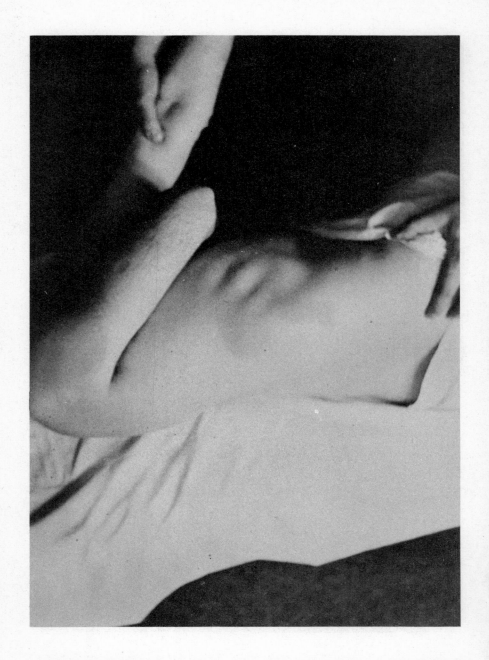

TORSO IS FLEXED PARTIALLY, THEN LATERALLY FLEXED AND ROTATED TO LOCK ARTICULATIONS. THIS GIVES A SLIGHT LIFT TO SACRUM THAT MUST BE CARRIED POS-TERO*SUPERIORLY, PARALLEL TO THE ARTICULAR SURFACE.

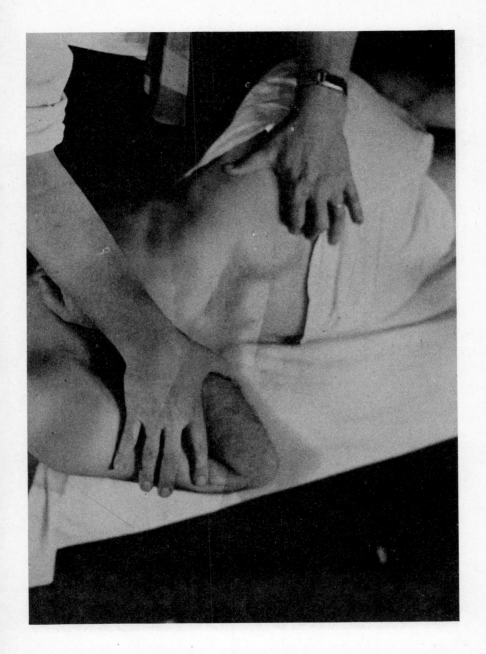

PRESSURE ON SHOULDER PROTECTS SPINAL ARTICULATIONS
WHILE ILIUM IS BROUGHT ANTERIORLY AND INFERIORLY.

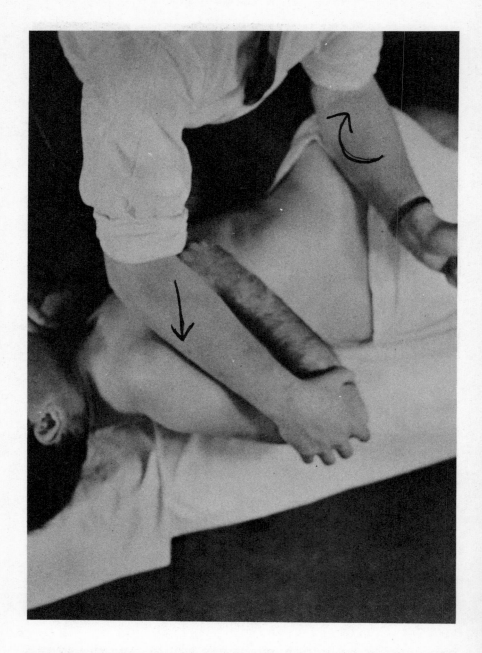

CORRECTIVE FORCE IS APPLIED WITH THE PADDED MUSCU-
LAR PART OF PHYSICIAN'S FORE-ARM, JUST BELOW THE
CREST OF ILIUM.

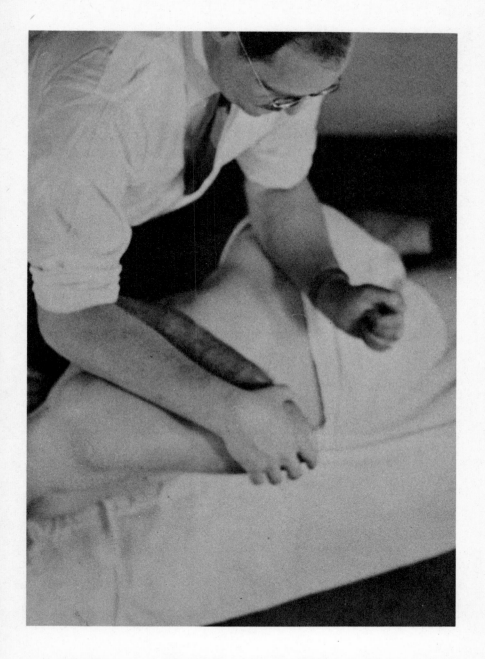

ALL MOTION IS CONSUMED- ANTAGONISTIC TENSION HELD
MOMENTARILY; THEN A THRUST IS ADDED, IF NECESSARY,
TO THE ILIUM, CARRYING IT ANTERO-INFERIORLY.

FLEXED SACRUM

CHUG TECHNIQUE

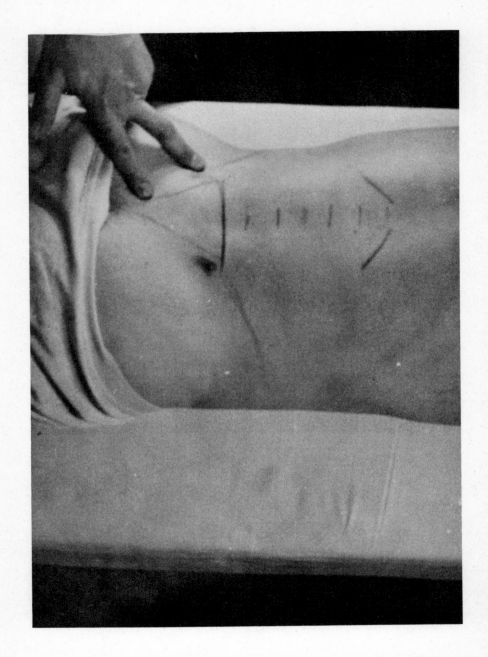

CHUG TECHNIQUE - PATIENT PRONE - PILLOW UNDER PEL-
VIS. PALPATING PROMINENT POSTERIOR SUPERIOR ILIAC
SPINE AND DEEPENED SACRAL GROOVE.

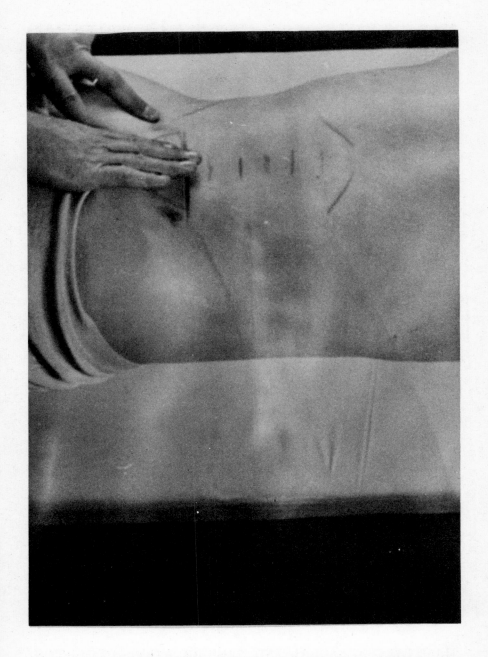

ILLUSTRATING POSITION OF SACRUM IN TORSION.

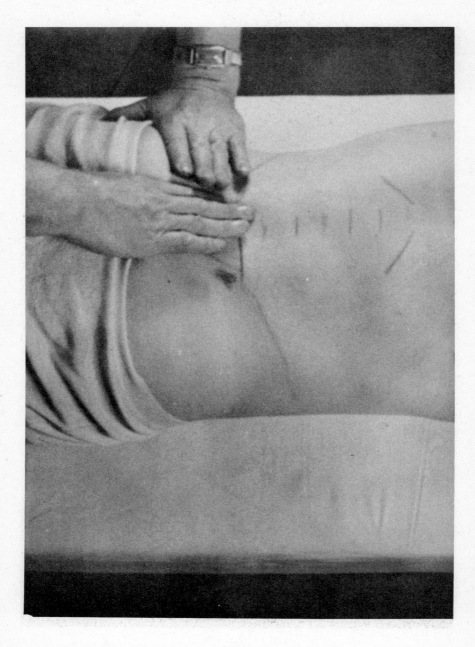

ILLUSTRATING SACRAL AND ILIAL RELATIONS IN TORSION.

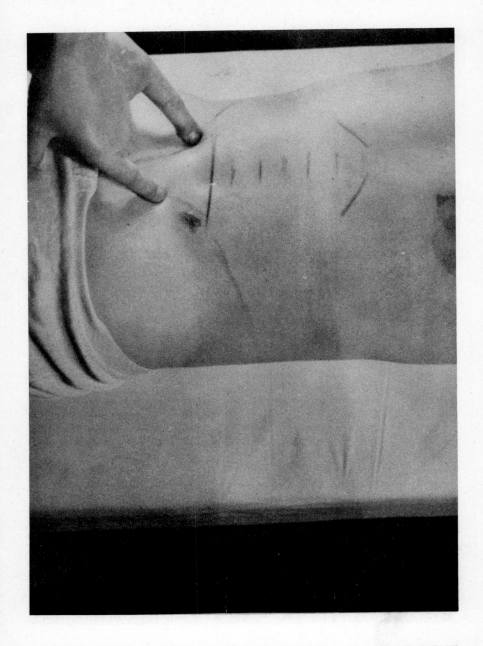

PALPATING TWO POINTS OF CONTACT - (1) PROMINENT
POSTERIOR SUPERIOR ILIAC SPINE ON FLEXED SACRAL SIDE;
(2) PROMINENT SACRUM ON EXTENDED SACRAL SIDE.

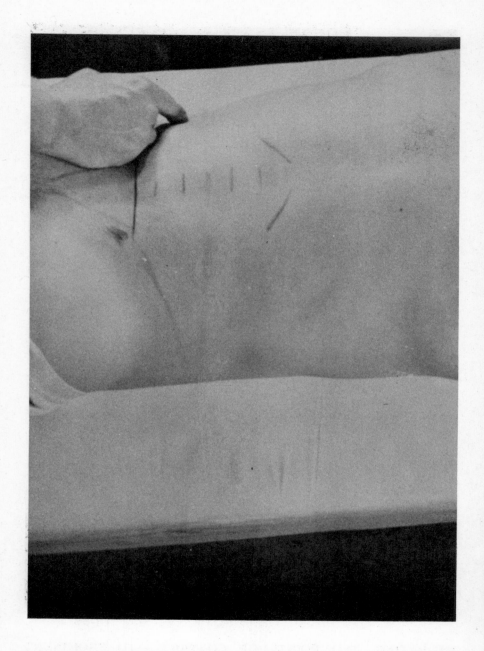

ILLUSTRATING DIRECTION OF FORCE TO BE APPLIED TO ILIUM.

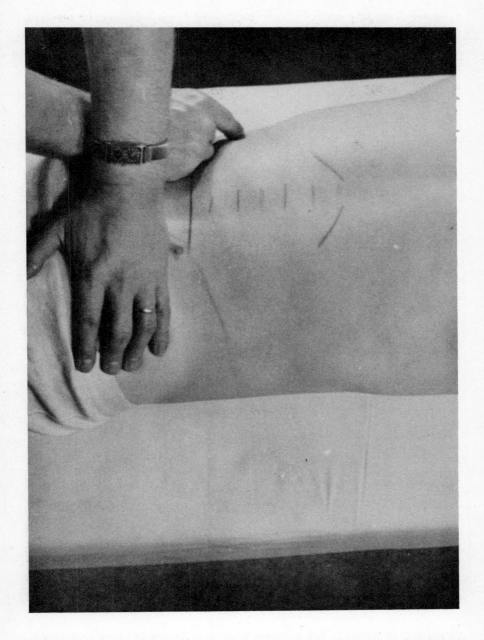

ADDING COUNTER AND SEPARATING FORCE TO EXTENDED
SACRAL SIDE.

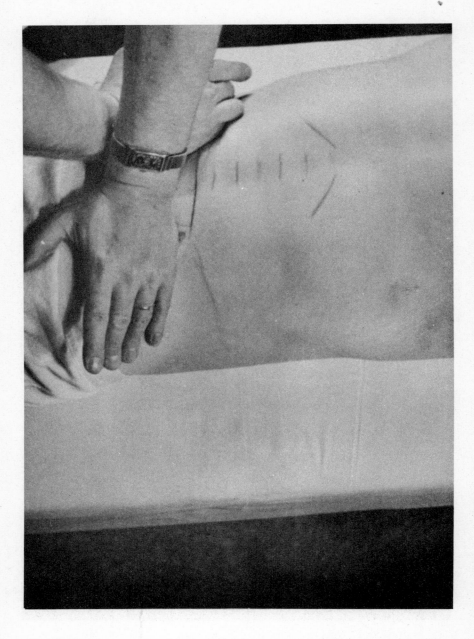

WEIGHT IS ADDED TO THE EXTENDED ARMS - APPROXIMATE-
LY 50 LBS.

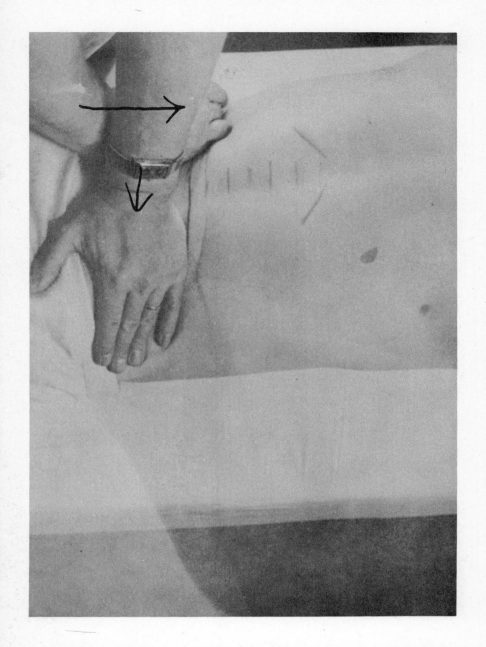

ADDITIONAL 10 OR 15 LBS. IS SUDDENLY APPLIED, HANDS
SEPARATING FROM EACH OTHER, TO SPRING SACRO-ILIAC
ARTICULATION APART AND THEN IN THE SPECIFIC DIREC-
TION FOR CORRECTION.

FLEXED SACRUM

HEAVY TRACTION WITH COUNTERFORCE

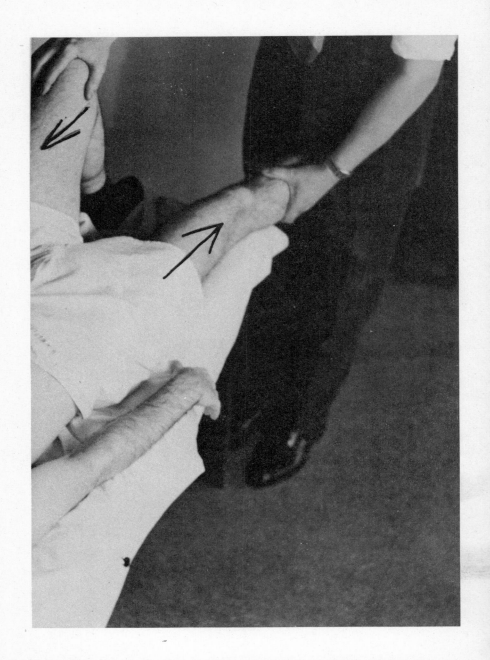

CEPHALIC FORCE DIRECTED WITH HANDS ON KNEE ON EX-
TENDED SACRAL SIDE. CAUDAL FORCE QUICKLY APPLIED
WITH BODY THRUST ON FLEXED SACRAL SIDE.

FLEXED SACRUM

LEG LEVERAGE TECHNIQUES

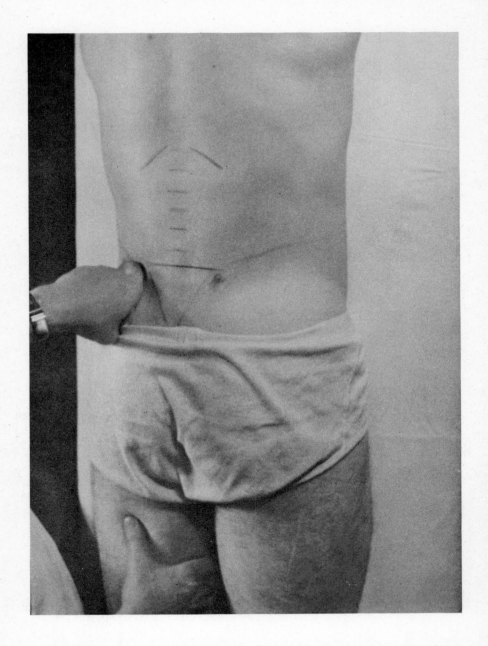

LEG LEVERAGE TECHNIQUE TO BE USED WITH EXTREME
CAUTION, NOT TRULY RECOMMENDED FOR CORRECTION.
ILLUSTRATING DIRECTION OF FORCE TO BE APPLIED TO
ILIUM.

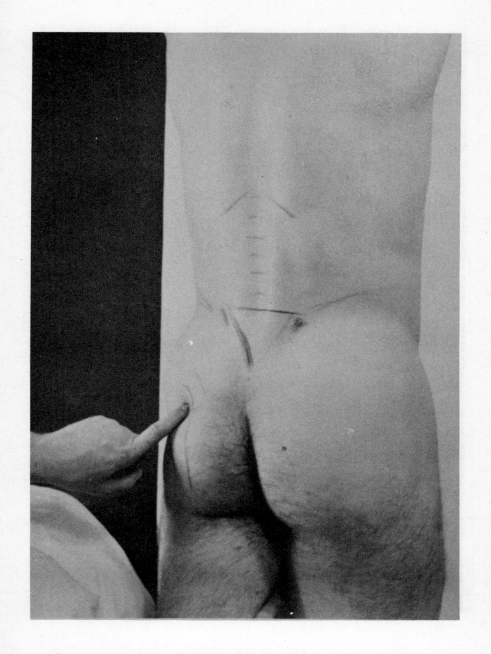

HIP JOINT AND FEMUR TO BE USED AS A LEVER

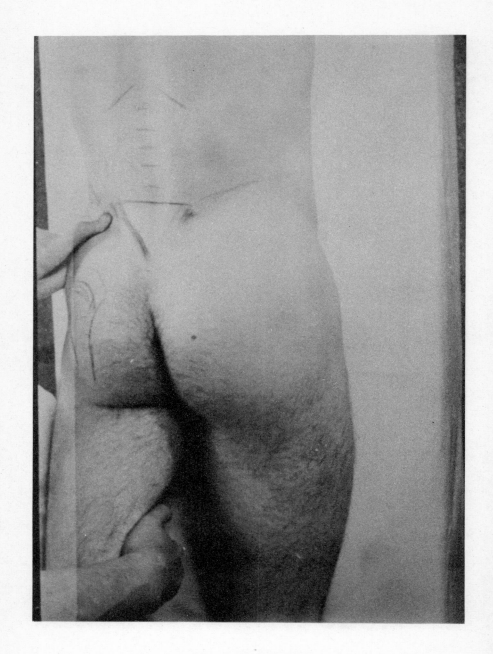

LEG IS EXTENDED

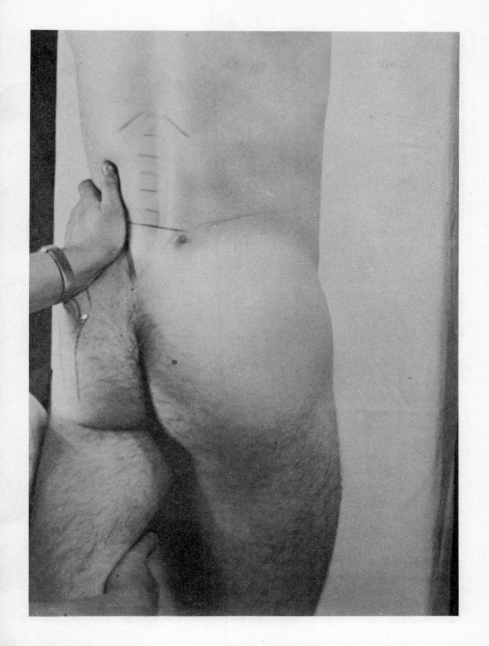

LEG EXTENDED COMPLETELY, COUNTER FORCE APPLIED
TO ILIUM.

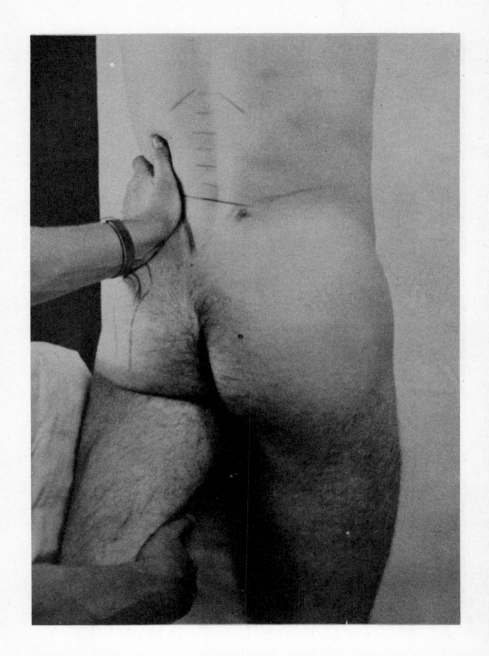

THRUST IS CAUTIOUSLY APPLIED - HYPEREXTENDING FEMUR
AND FORCING ILIUM ANTERIORLY FROM THE FLEXED SA-
CRUM.

FLEXED SACRUM - UNILATERAL OR BILATERAL TECHNIQUES FOR CORRECTION

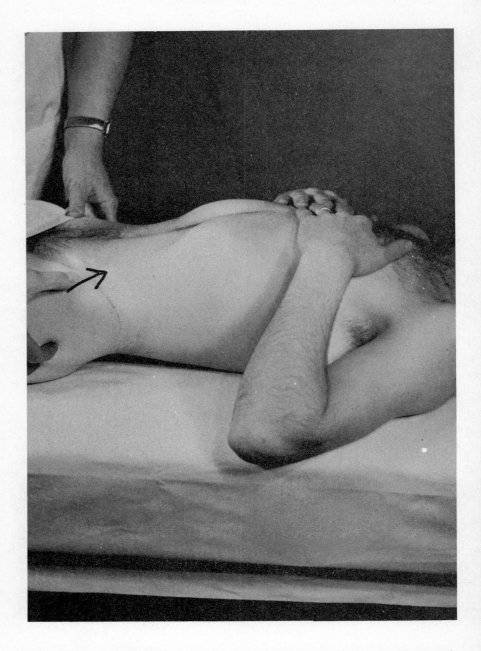

ILLUSTRATING CEPHALIC AND PROMINENT ANTERIOR SUPER-
IOR ILIAC SPINE ON FLEXED SACRAL SIDE IN SACRAL TOR-
SION.

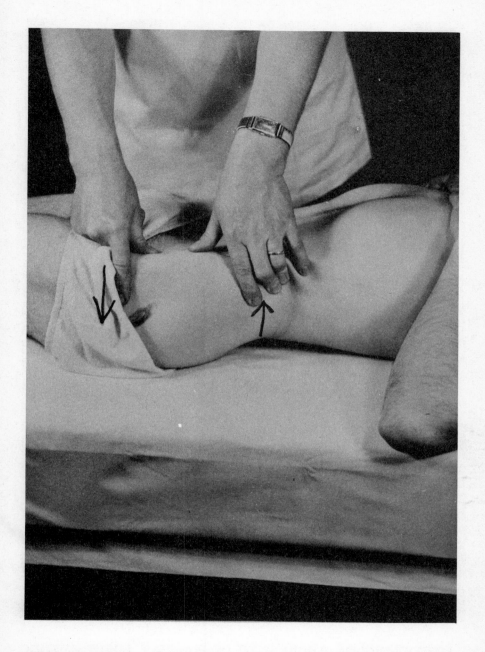

ILLUSTRATING DIRECTION OF CORRECTIVE FORCE ROTATING
ILIUM ANTERIORLY AROUND THE SECOND SACRAL SEGMENT.

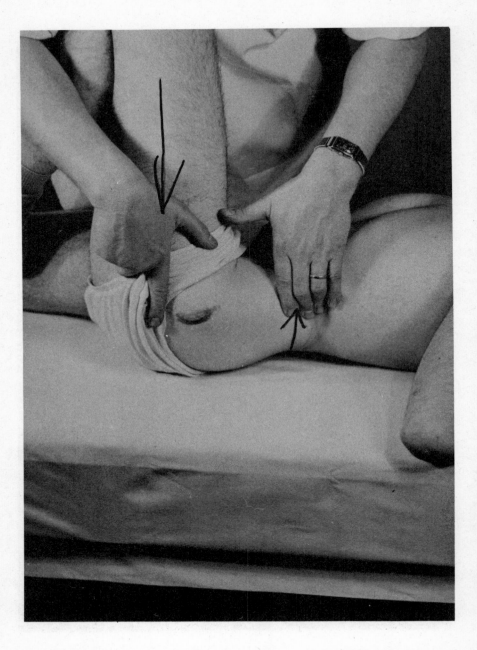

POSITIONING OF THIGH WITH CORRECTIVE FORCE, MOVING
ACETABULUM CAUDAD BELOW SECOND SACRAL SEGMENT.

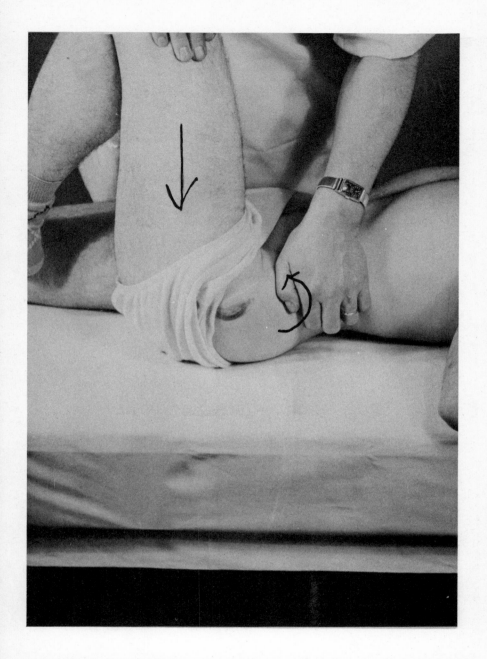

CORRECTIVE THRUST APPLIED DOWNWARD TO CORRECT
MAL-ALIGNMENT AND RESTORE MOTION.

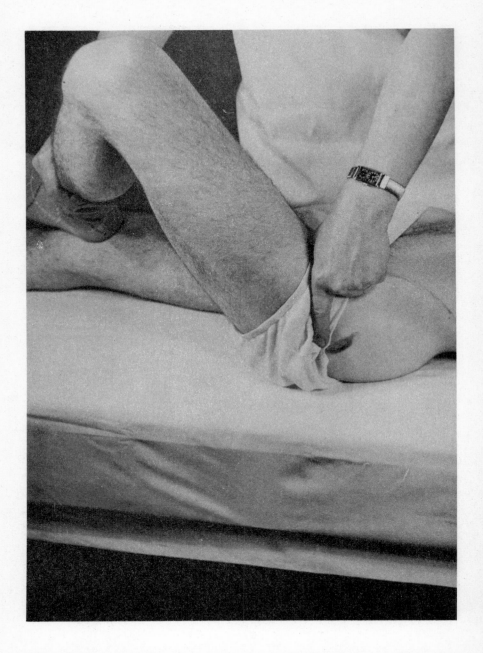

LEG LEVERAGE, RELATIVE LEG LENGTHENING TECHNIQUE FOR FLEXED SACRAL SIDE.

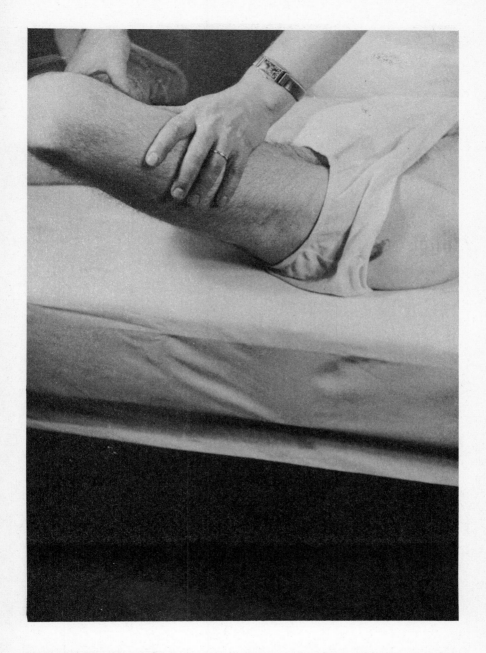

LEG ROCKED LATERALLY - WEIGHT OF LEG PULLS ILIUM
FORWARD THRU DOWNWARD FORCE AT ACETABULUM.

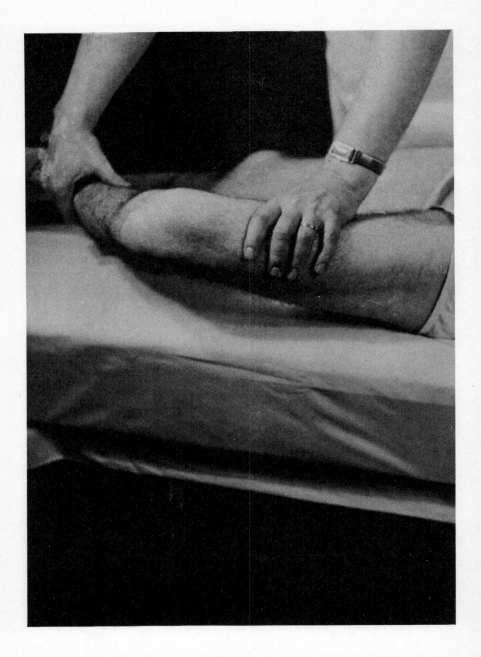

FORCE INCREASED BY ABDUCTION AND STRAIGHTENING OF LEG AND THIGH.

EXTENDED SACRUM
LATERAL
TECHNIQUES

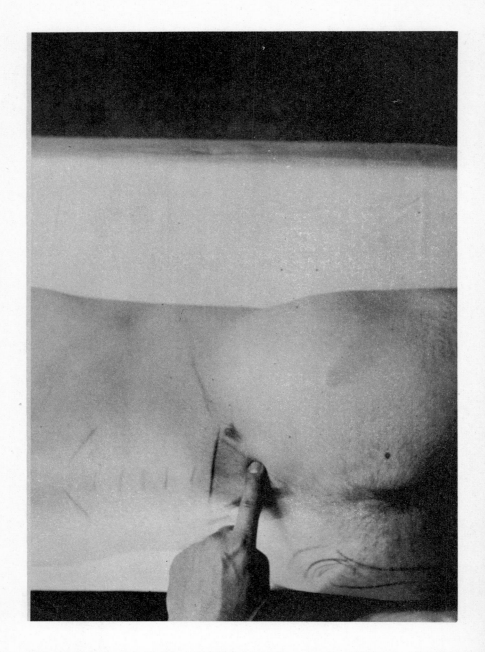

PALPATION OF PROMINENT SIDE OF SACRUM ON EXTENDED
SIDE OF TORSION TOWARD THAT SIDE.

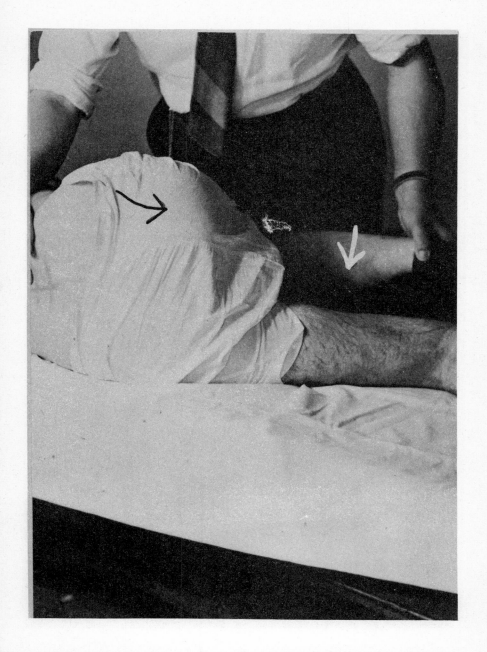

LEG DROPPED OFF TABLE TO AID POSTERIOR ROTATION
OF ILIUM.

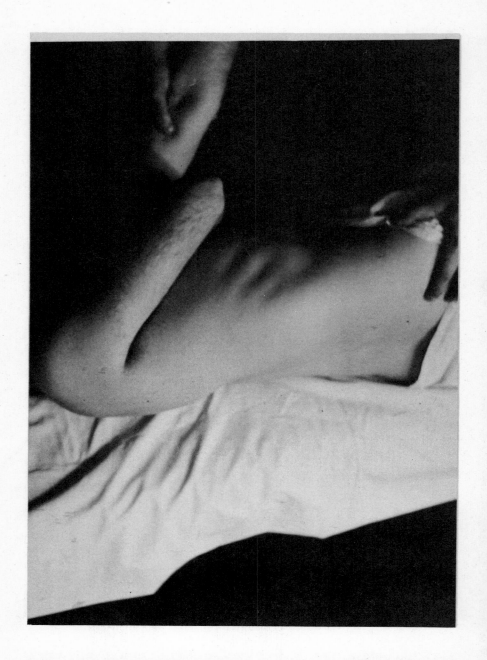

SHOULDER IS <u>NOT</u> ROTATED, FOR A SPINAL ROTATION WOULD PULL POSTERIORLY ON THE SACRAL SIDE ALREADY IN EXTENSION LESION.

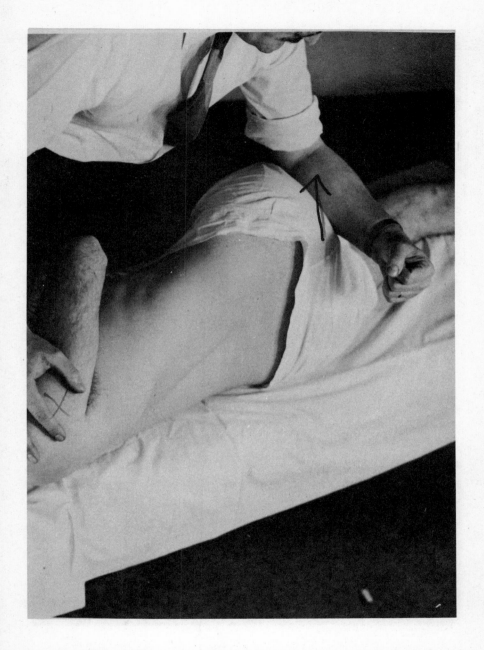

SHOULDER IS HELD BY CEPHALIC HAND. FOREARM PULLS
ISCHIAL TUBEROSITY FORWARD TO POINT OF TENSION.

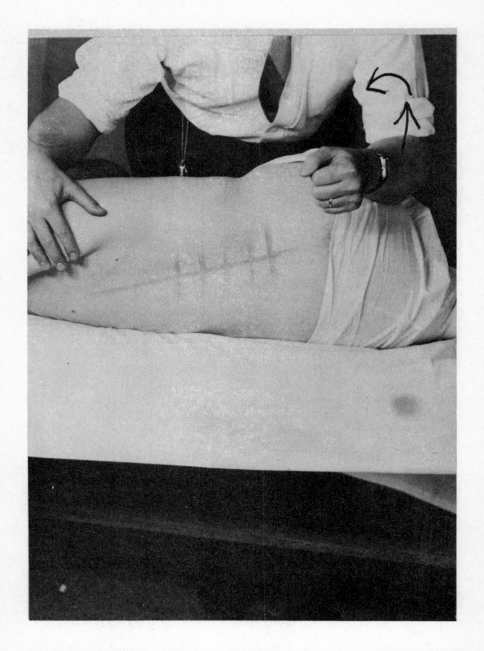

MAINTAINING FORWARD PULL ON ISCHIUM, THE FORCE IS
BENT CEPHALICALLY AND CARRIED LONGITUDINALLY UP-
WARD UNTIL TENSION IS PRODUCED.

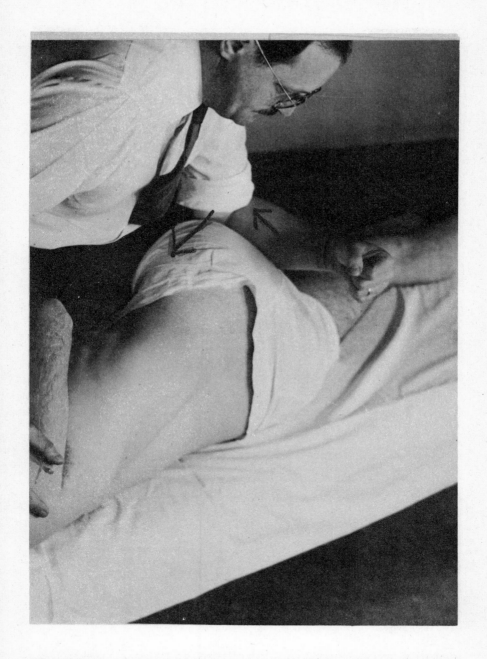

CORRECTIVE FORCE IS SUDDEN AND IS DIRECTLY CEPHALAD.
NO COUNTERFORCE SHOULD BE APPLIED TO SHOULDER.

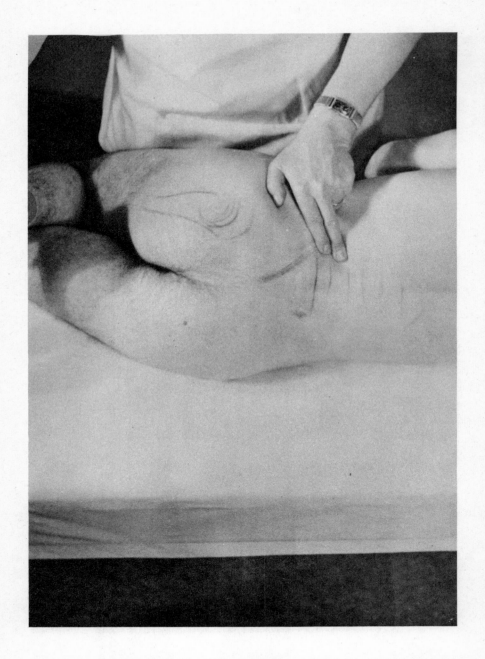

WOBBLE TECHNIQUE FOR EXTENDED SACRUM - APPLIED ON
THAT SIDE OF A SACRAL TORSION AND ON BOTH SIDES IN
BILATERALLY EXTENDED SACRUM. THIS IS A MEDIOCRE PIECE
OF TECHNIQUE. PALPATING THE DECREASED PROMINENCE
OF THE POSTERIOR SUPERIOR ILIAC SPINE AND THE SHAL-
LOWED SACRAL GROOVE OF THE EXTENDED SACRAL SIDE.

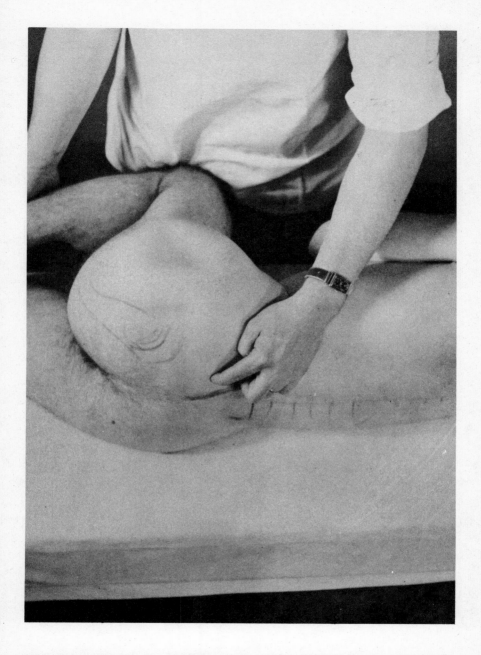

PATIENT'S KNEE IS FORCED CEPHALICALLY TO EXERT HAM-
STRING MUSCLE PULL AND FORCE ILIUM POSTERIORLY ON
THE EXTENDED SACRUM.

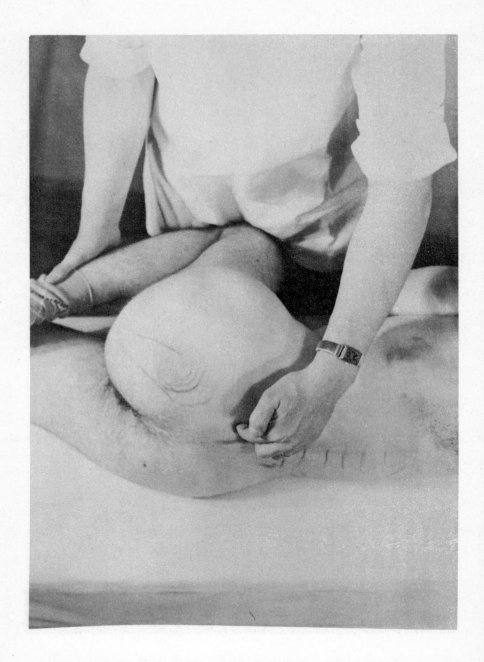

FINGERS ARE FORCED ONTO THE UPPER SEGMENTS OF THE
SACRUM ON THE EXTENDED SIDE, DIRECTING THAT SIDE OF
SACRUM ANTERIORLY AND INFERIORLY PARALLEL TO THE
PLANE OF THE ARTICULATION.

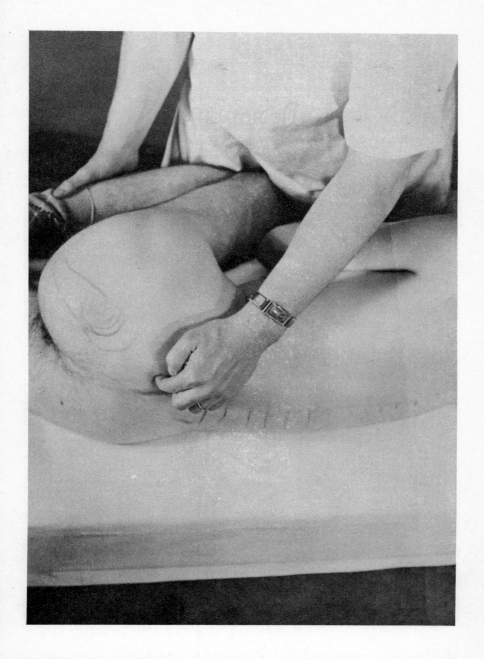

PATIENT'S FEMUR IS STRONGLY FLEXED ON THE ILIUM;
FORCE RESISTED BY FINGERS PULLING ANTERIORLY ON EX-
TENDED SACRUM.

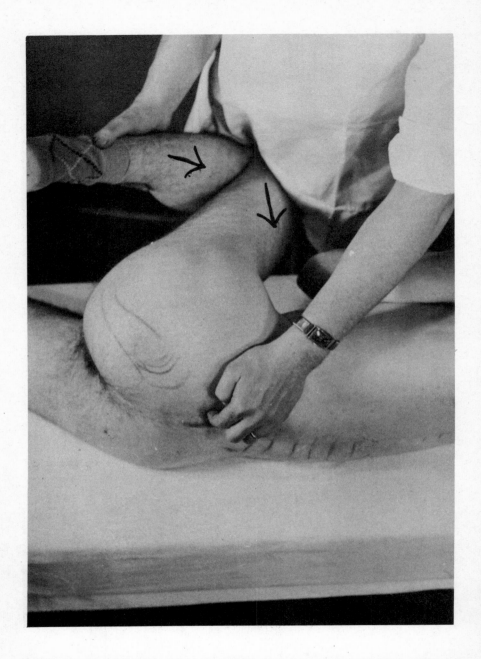

LEG IS WOBBLED IN ADDUCTION AND ABDUCTION WHILE
TENSION IS TRANSMITTED THRU HIP JOINT TO ILIUM TO
ROCK POSTERIORLY ON THE POSTERIOR OR EXTENDED SA-
CRUM. THIS TECHNIQUE, OBVIOUSLY, CAN INJURE THE HIP
JOINT IF TOO VIGOROUSLY APPLIED.

EXTENDED SACRUM

HAMSTRING PULL

TECHNIQUE

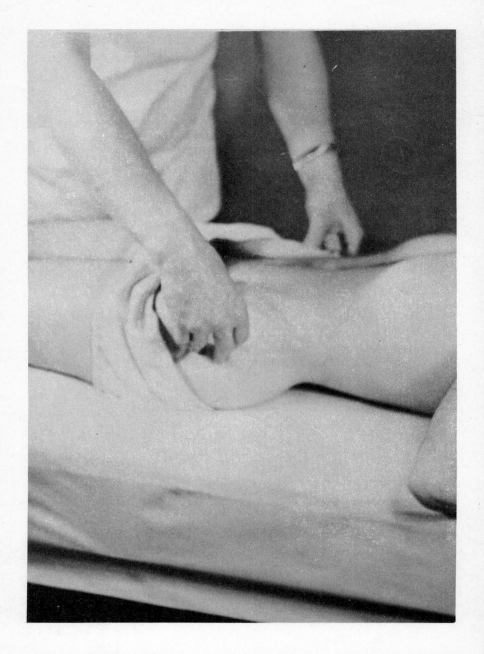

COMPARING PROMINENCE OF ANTERIOR SUPERIOR ILIAC SPINES FOR CEPHALIC OR CAUDAD SHIFT, AS IN SACRAL TORSION.

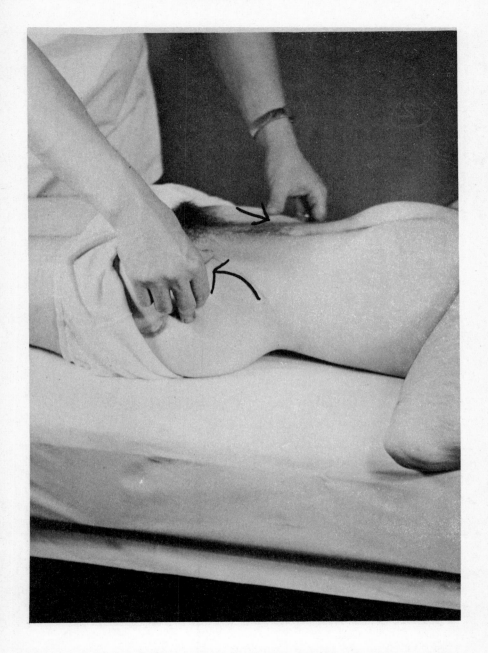

CAUDAL SHIFT AND LESSENED PROMINENCE ON SIDE OF EX-
TENDED SACRUM, RELATIVELY LENGTHENING LEG.

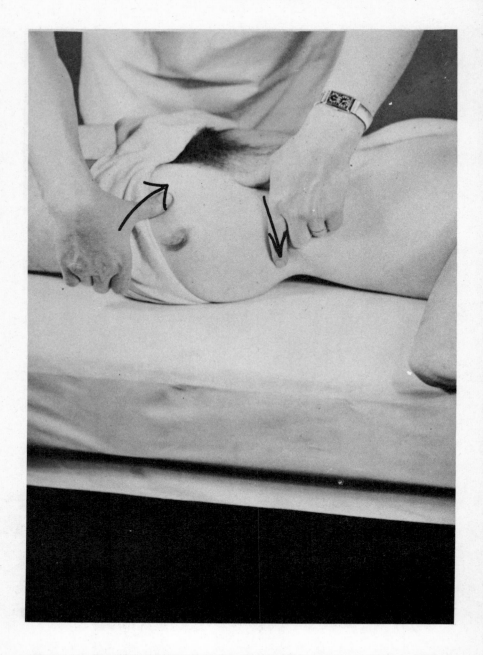

INDICATING CORRECTIVE DIRECTION ON ILIUM ON EXTEND-
ED SACRAL OR ANTERIOR INNOMINATE SIDE.

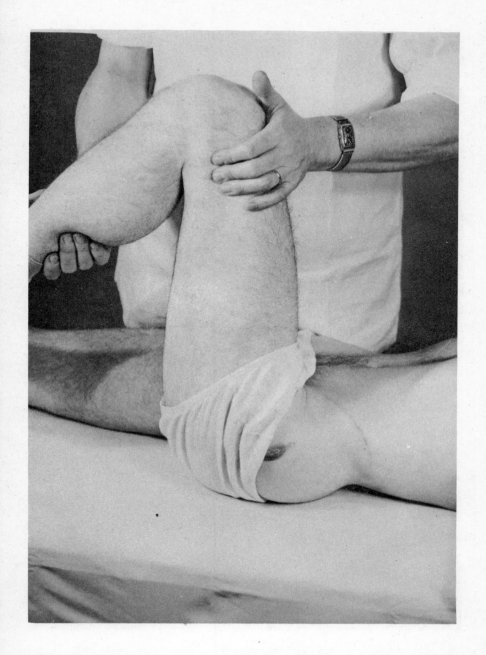

BEGINNING OF LEG TRACTION CORRECTION TO ROCK ILIUM
POSTERIORLY ON SACRUM.

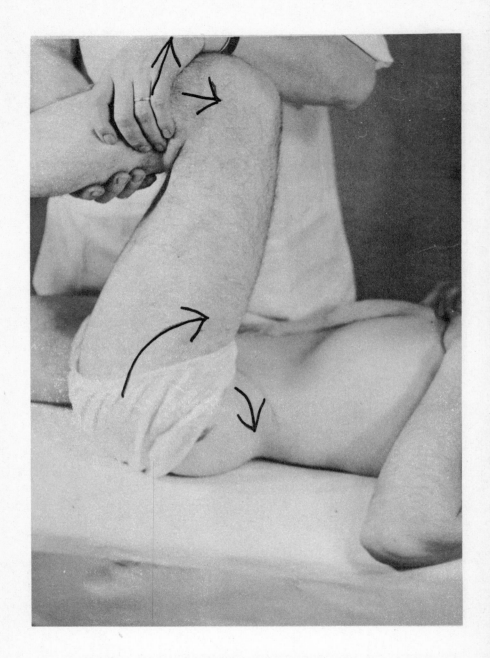

LEG FLEXED ON THIGH, THIGH FLEXED ON PELVIS.

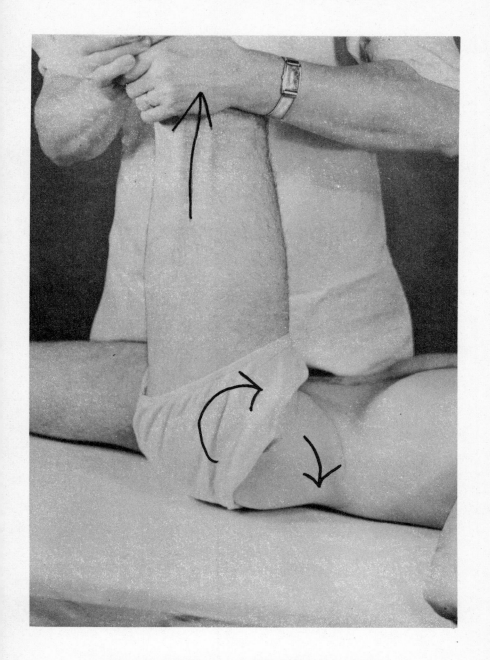

SUDDEN THRUST OF TRACTION ON LEG.

EXTENDED SACRUM
LEG LEVERAGE
TECHNIQUES

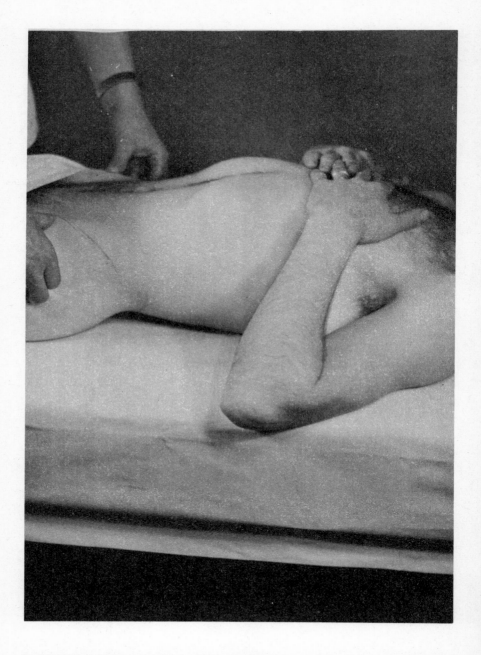

ILLUSTRATING CAUDALLY SHIFTED ANTERIOR SUPERIOR
ILIAC SPINE ON EXTENDED SACRAL SIDE.

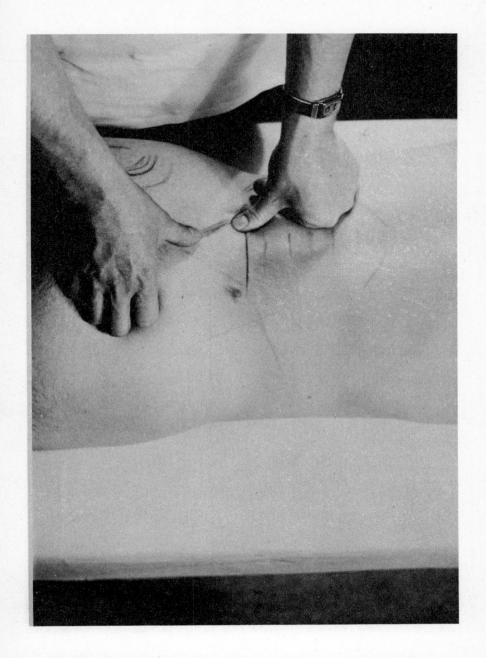

ILLUSTRATING DEEPENED SACRAL GROOVE ON OPPOSITE OR
FLEXED SIDE IN SACRAL TORSION.

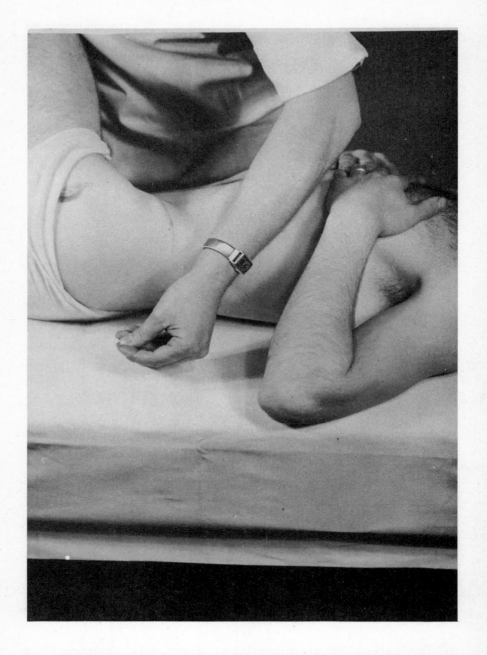

FINGERS ARE BUNCHED TO CREATE A PROMINENCE TO PLACE UNDER THE SACRAL TOP ON THE EXTENDED SIDE.

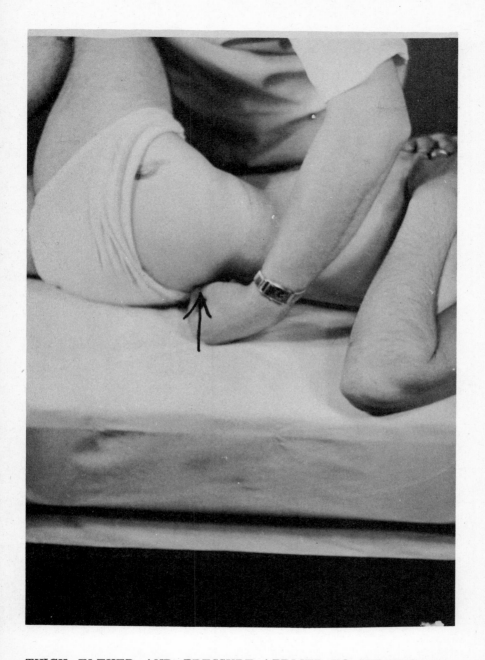

THIGH FLEXED AND PRESSURE APPLIED TO SUPERIOR SA-
CRAL SEGMENT ON EXTENDED SACRAL SIDE.

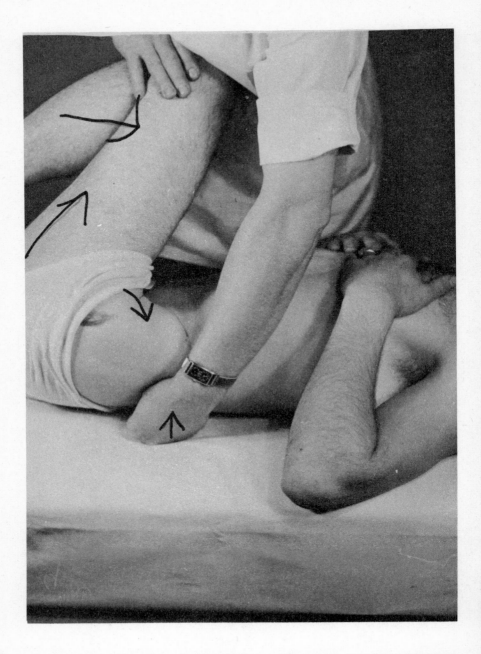

THIGH IS STRONGLY FLEXED. HAMSTRING PULL FORCING
ILIUM POSTERIORLY ON EXTENDED SIDE OF SACRUM.

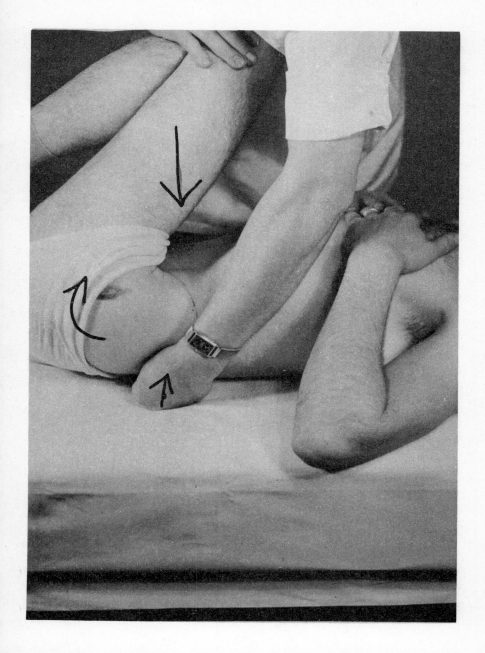

INCREASED PRESSURE ON THIGH ACCENTUATES PRESSURE
ON FINGERS CARRYING SACRUM ANTERIORLY INTO FLEXION.

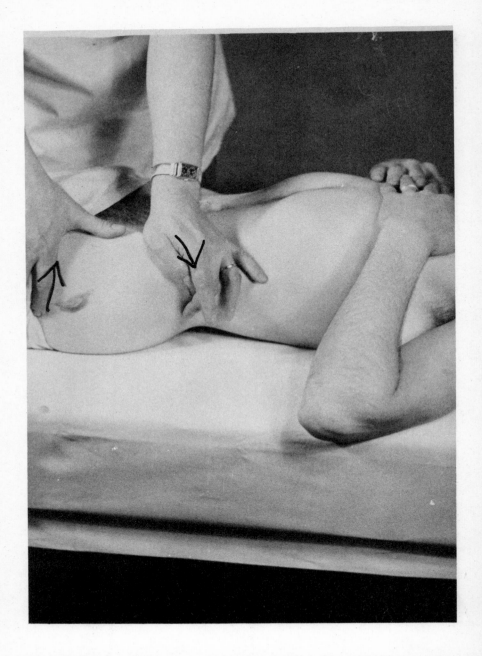

ALTERNATE TECHNIC. ILLUSTRATING DIRECTION OF COR-
RECTIVE FORCE.

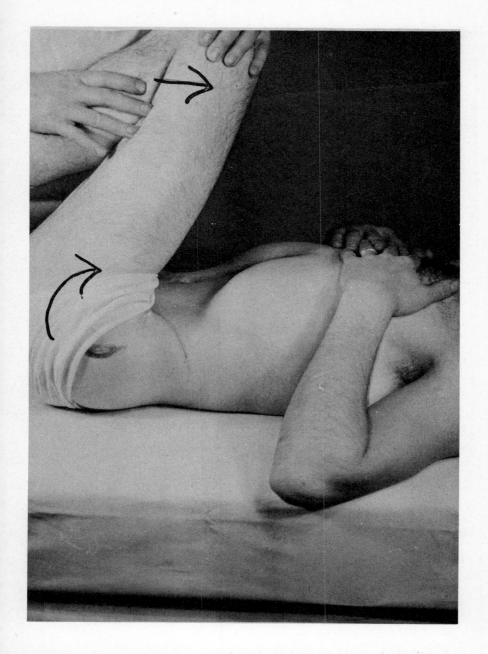

LEG FLEXED TO PRODUCE HAMSTRING PULL AND ROCK IL-
IUM POSTERIORLY ON SACRUM.

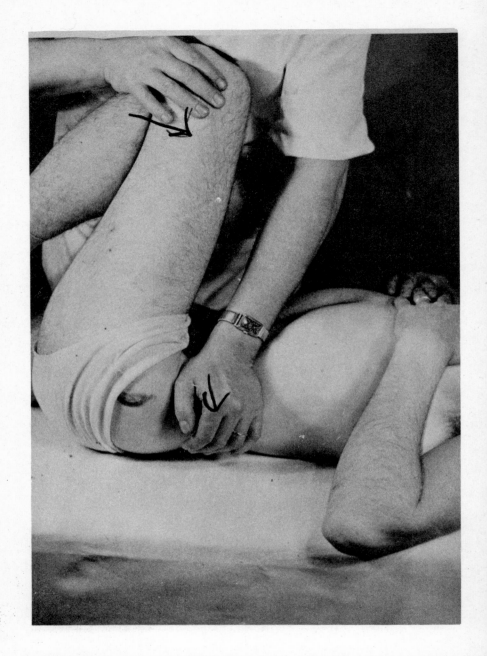

ADDUCTION AND FLEXION ROCKING OF THE THIGH SHOULD
MOVE THE ILIUM POSTERIORLY. COMBINED PRESSURE ON
THE ANTERIOR SUPERIOR ILIAC SPINE MAY BE USED.

SACRAL TORSION
BILATERAL TECHNIQUE

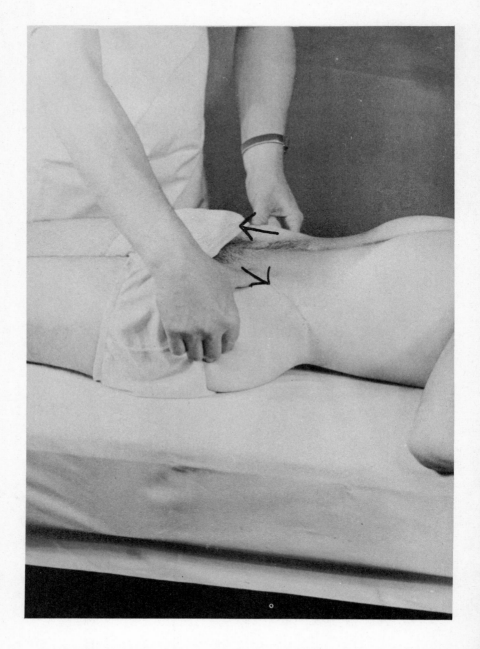

ILLUSTRATING ILIUM SHIFT IN PELVIC OR SACRAL TORSION.

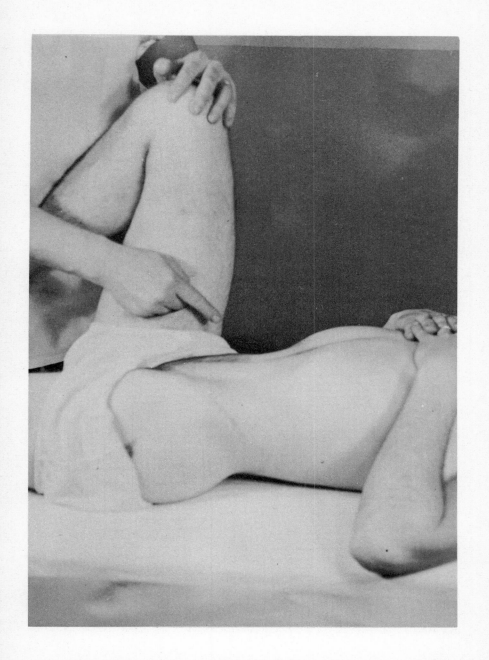

CORRECTIVE DIRECTION ON EXTENDED SACRAL SIDE.

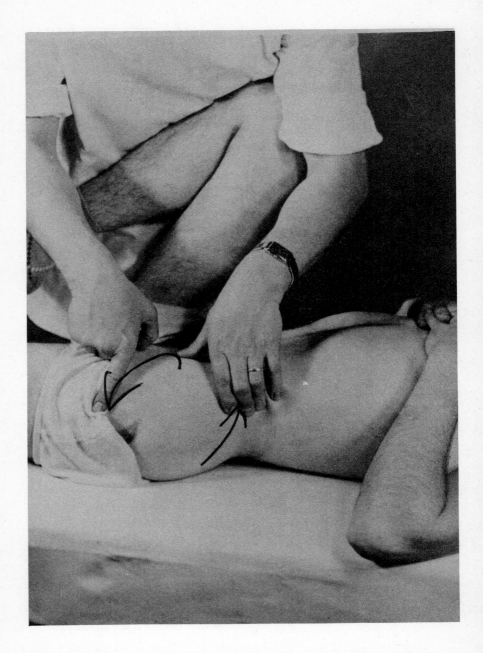

CORRECTIVE DIRECTION ON FLEXED SACRAL SIDE.

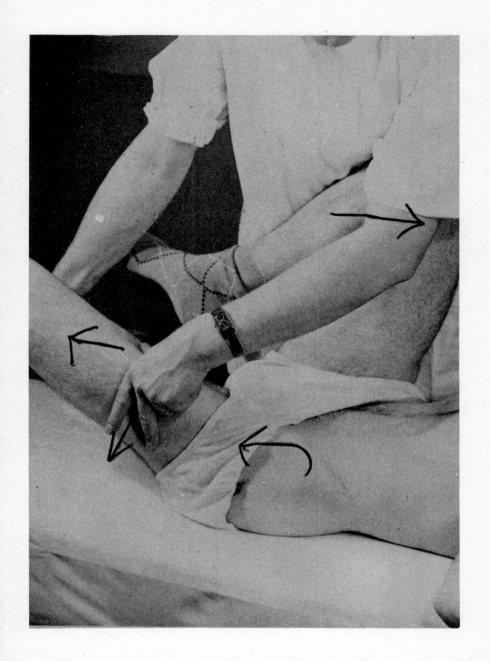

BILATERAL LEG LEVERAGE FORCES TO MOVE ILIA ON
FIXED SACRUM.

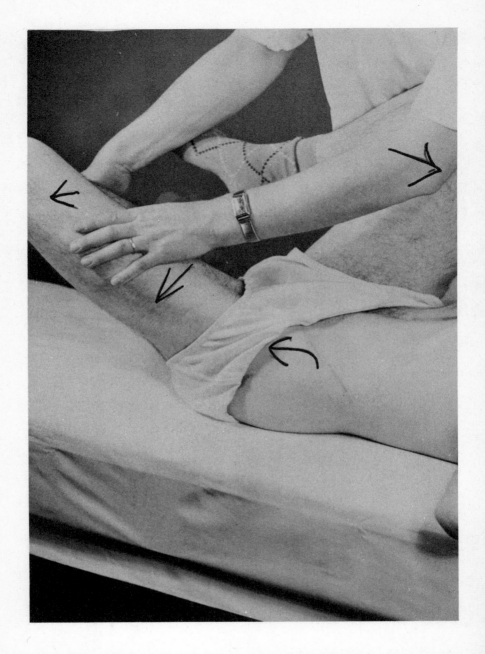

FORCES INCREASED. LEG ON FLEXED SIDE IS ROCKED TO
MOVE ILIUM ANTERIORLY.

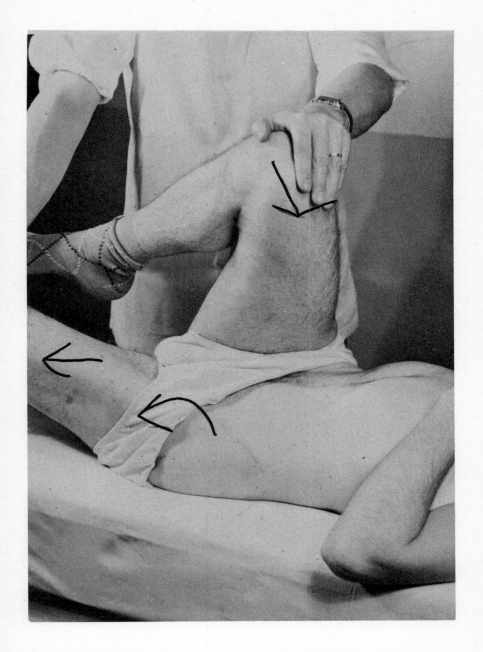

LEGS MAY BE ROCKED WITHOUT APPRECIABLE FORCE.

PUBIC

TECHNIQUES

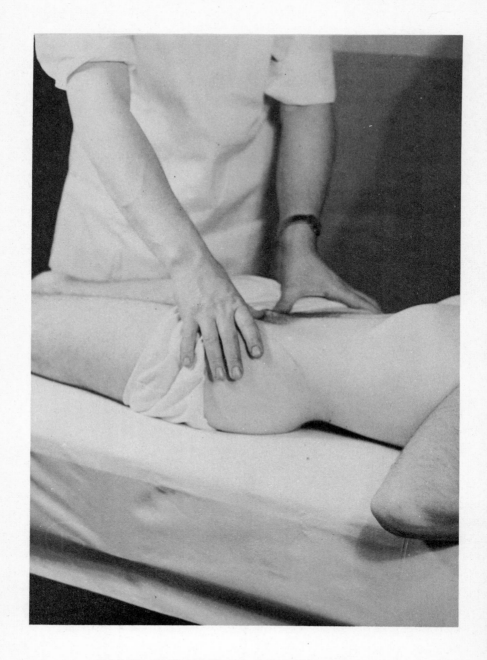

FORCE DESIGNED TO RE-ALIGN PUBES.

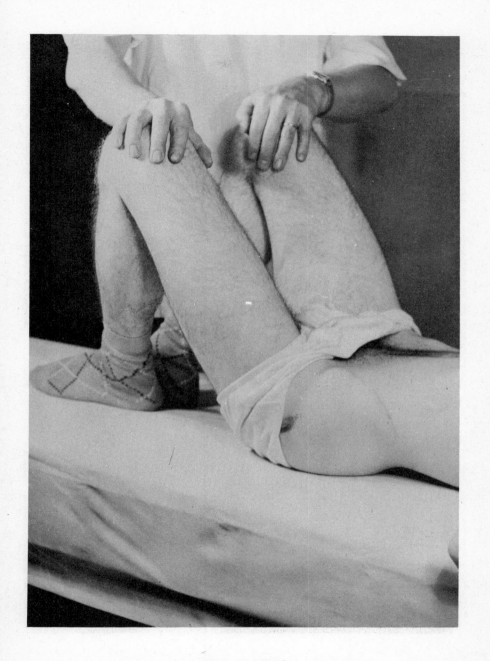

LEGS FLEXED

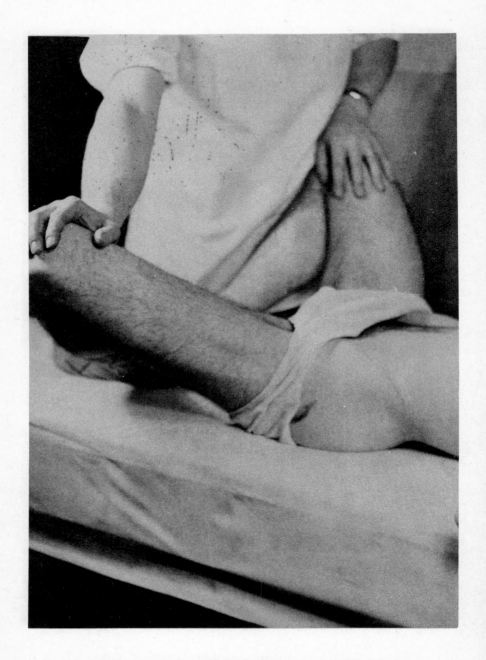

KNEES FORCED APART WITH SLIGHT THRUST.

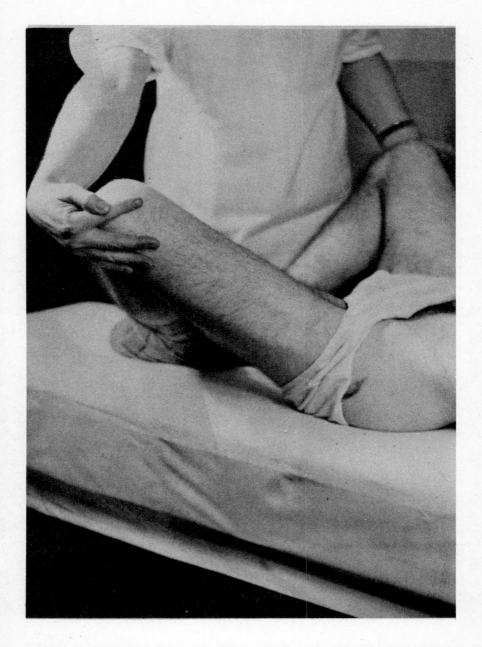

HANDS MAY RESIST PATIENT'S ABDUCTION. THEN SUDDEN-
LY REMOVE THE HANDS. WEIGHT OF LEGS WILL SEPARATE
AND RE-ALIGN PUBES.

LUMBAR AREA

CONGENITAL ANOMALIES

At the lumbo-sacral area appears an array of congenital anomalies that are encountered with perplexing frequency. Their presence necessitates early and accurate diagnosis. Treatment is not conducive to great variation. The following outline is a list of the common ones associated with many acute and most recurrent low back syndromes.

1. Leg length difference and its cephalic effect.
2. Lumbo-sacral angle:
   (a) Pseudospondylolisthesis
   (b) Straight or poker type spine.
3. Lumbar index varying from 1-1/2 inches.
4. Spina bifida occulta
5. Assimilation phenomena
   (a) Cephalic-lumbarization of sacrum
   (b) Caudal-sacralization of lumbar area.
6. Numerical variation- supra and infra numerary vertebra or /and ribs.
7. Hemi-vertebrae
8. Anomalous enlargements
   (a) Spinous processes (becoming weight bearing)
   (b) Alar transverse processes (may articulate with each other, the sacrum or ilium).
9. Spondylolysis
10. Spondylolisthesis
11. Schmorl's Nodes
12. Anomalous facets.

The management of spondylolisthesis may require fusion if anti-gravity cast or brace is effective for a period of time.

The remaining of the above are rarely ever markedly improved by surgery, but require manipulation, judiciously and frequently applied, along with belts, braces, occupational and postural change.

Leg length has been discussed in the hip joint area.

Lumbo-sacral angle has been determined as a mechanical necessity at 37-1/2º.

Lumbar index must be 1-1/2 inches. Lumbar index and lumbo-sacral angle usually undergo identical variations from the normal and are susceptible to the same treatment.

Heel height and sole thickness are mechanical aids. The higher the heel and the lower the sole, the greater will become the lumbo-sacral angle and the lumbar index. Lowering the heel and if necessary thickening the soles will reduce those measurements. Increased gluteal muscle tone will antagonize the psoas units and reduce the lumbar index and the lumbo-sacral angle.

IT IS A MECHANICAL CERTAINTY THAT THE SACRUM MUST BE LEVEL AT ITS LATERAL ASPECTS, AND THE LUMBO-SACRAL ANGLE AND LUMBAR INDEX AS STIPULATED IF ONE EXPECTS TO HAVE ANY VALUABLE THERAPEUTIC EFFECT ON THE PATIENT AT THAT AREA OR ABOVE IT, SOMATIC OR VISCERAL.

LUMBAR AREA

The lumbosacral facets face each other on a plane that diverges postero-laterally at 37 to 45 degrees. This divergence permits a moderate amount of rotation.

Therefore in fifth lumbar lesions in addition to hypertonicity of muscle and pain there is often easily detected spinous process deviation, evidence of rotation along with lateral flexion.

Lesions of the remaining lumbar articulations possess much less rotation, inasmuch as the articulations face each other across an Anteroposterior Plan. Rotation readily approximates these facets, hence torsional forces are usually traumatic in the lumbar spine as in the knee joint where rotation is almost non-physiological.

LUMBAR LESIONS

A facet or segment may be lesioned and held in any position. The point of importance from a diagnostic approach is not so much the malalignment but the impaired mobility. Motion is essential for return circulation. When motion is absent there is an inevitable impairment of nervous and lymphatic return with its subsequent inflammatory reaction in tissue.

Lumbar lesions may find the vertebra above restricted in the position of bilateral flexion, bilateral extension, lateral flexion with rotation, or rarely in the middle of its range of motion. In the latter all the diagnostic signs of lesion pathology will be present except malalignment of parts. Outlined below are the physical findings of the above lesions.

	BILATERAL EXTENSION	BILATERAL FLEXION
Front of body of vertebra	Elevated	Anterior and inferior
Back of body of vertebra	Postero-inferior	Antero-superior
Ant. ligament	Tight	Relaxed
Post. ligament	Relaxed	Tight
Disc compression	Posteriorly	Anteriorly
Facets	Segment above moved inferiorly on segment below.	Segment above moved anterior superiorly on segment below.
Transverse process	Approximates those below, restriction in area of approximation	Approximates one above. Restriction in area of separation.
Spinous process	Approximates one below, restriction in area of approximation. Less prominent	Approximates one above. Restriction in area of separation. More prominent

With either type will be present also the other signs of lesion pathology; impaired motion, muscle hypertonicity, pain and hyperesthesia, with evidence of the inflammatory change in the soft tissues segmentally related.

LATERAL FLEXION WITH ROTATION LESIONS

	EXTENDED FACET SIDE	FLEXED FACET SIDE
Body of vertebra on one below	Tilts downward. Rotates toward this side	Tilts upward. Rotates toward opposite side.
Facet	Overlaps or approx. as in extension	Separates; moves superiorly as in flexion.
Transverse Process	Approximates one below. Becomes more prominent.	Approximates one above. Becomes less prominent.
Spinous process	Shifts to convex side	Shifts toward this side.
Apparent curve	Concave side	Convex side.
Disc	Compressed	Annulus under tension
Ligaments	Relaxed	Tight
Muscle tissue	Hypertonic	Stretched.

Motion will be deficient. Lesions are predominantly unilateral and usually on the extended facet side. Accurate position diagnosis is essential so the correctional force will not stretch already traumatized tissues, but will carry the facet back thru its normal range of motion coincident with the plane of the articulation.

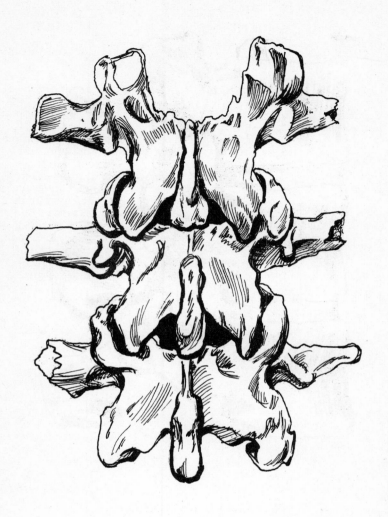

BILATERAL EXTENSION

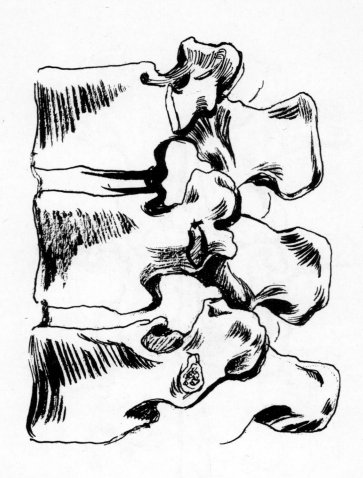

BILATERAL EXTENSION

LATERAL VIEW

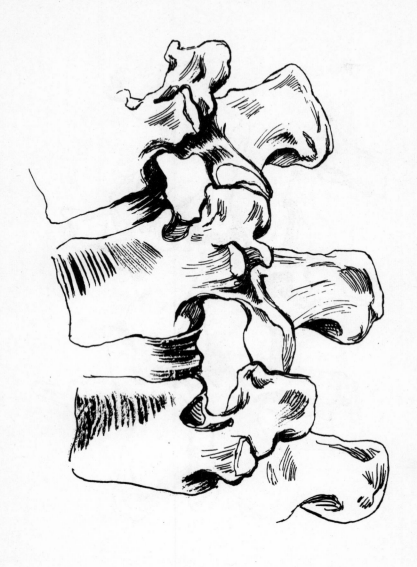

BILATERAL FLEXION

LATERAL VIEW

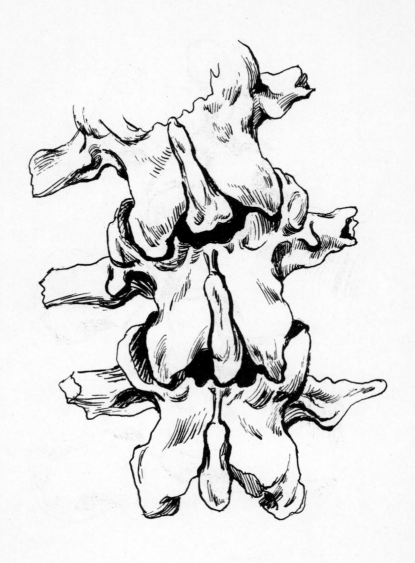

LATERAL FLEXION

WITH ROTATION

FLEXED FACET TECHNIQUES
LUMBAR AREA

FLEXED LUMBAR FACET
LATERAL TECHNIQUE

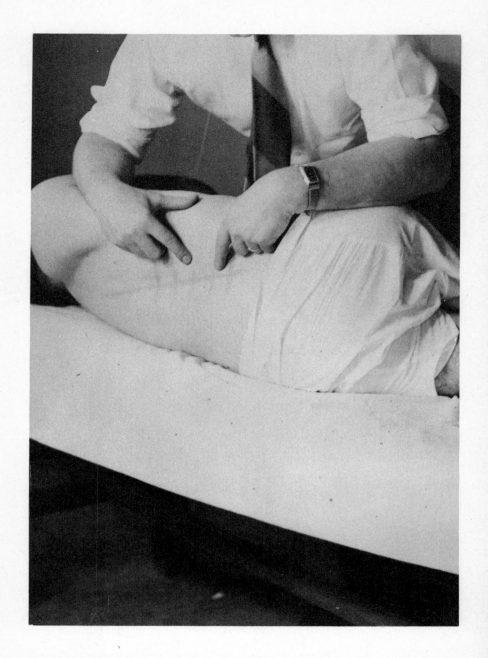

ILLUSTRATING FLEXED OR SEPARATED FACET. CONVEX
SIDE OF A CURVE. SIDE FROM WHICH LATERAL FLEXION
WITH ROTATION OF VERTEBRAL BODY TAKES PLACE.

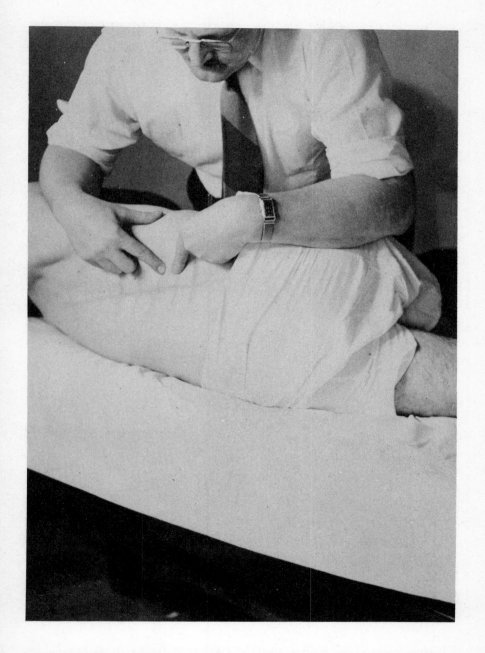

ILLUSTRATING REVERSAL OF POSITION, THE OBJECT OF
THE TECHNIQUE.

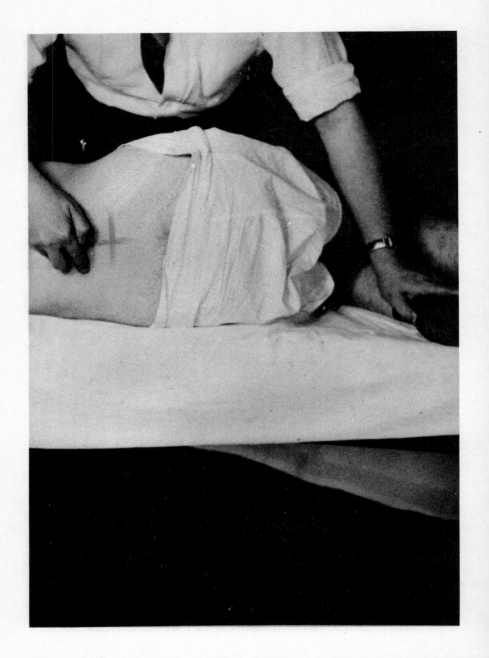

LOWER LEG IS FLEXED UNTIL TENSION IN THE DEPENDANT
MUSCULATURE ASCENDS TO THE INFERIOR OF THE TWO
SEGMENTS IN LESION.

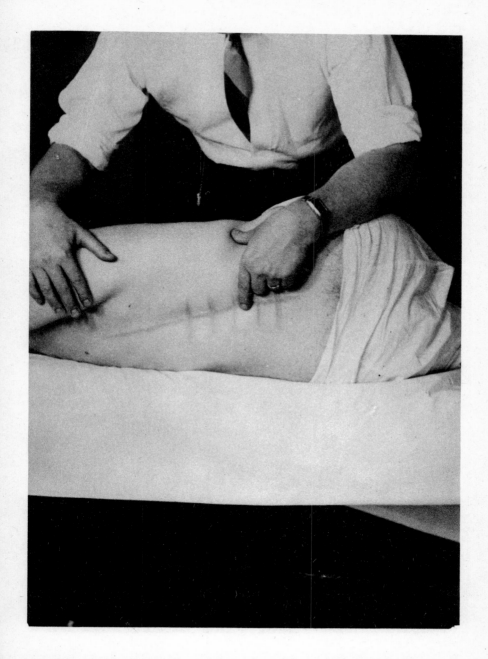

ROTATION OF SHOULDER AND LATERAL FLEXION WITH RO-
TATION OF SPINAL SEGMENTS DOWN TO UPPER OF THE
TWO SEGMENTS IN LESION. THIS PROTECTS THEM AGAINST
ASSUMPTION OF THE SUBSEQUENT CORRECTIVE FORCE.

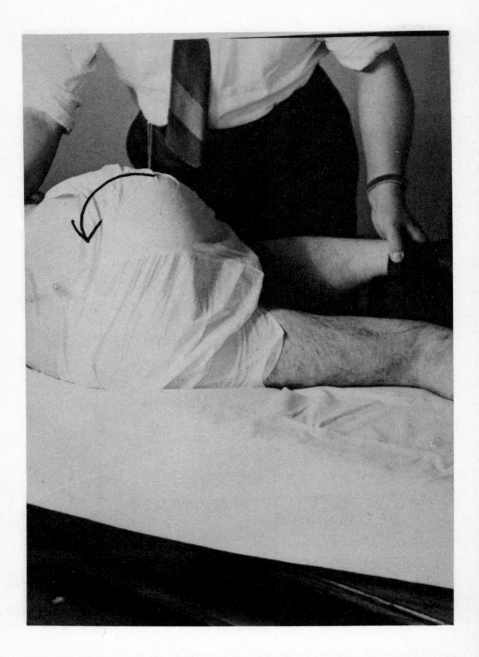

SINCE THIS TECHNIQUE REQUIRES THE ILIUM TO ROTATE POSTERIORLY, THE WEIGHT OF THE LEG BECOMES AN AD-VANTAGE, SO LEG IS DROPPED OFF THE TABLE.

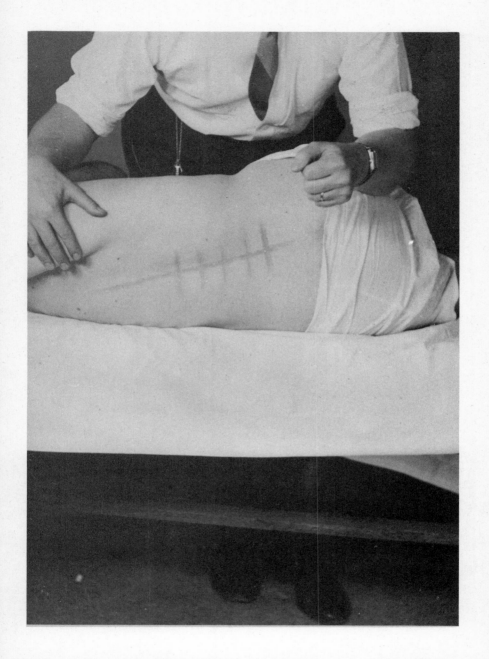

CEPHALIC ARM FIXES SHOULDER. CAUDAL ARM BRINGS
ISCHIAL TUBEROSITY ANTERIORLY AND SUPERIORLY.

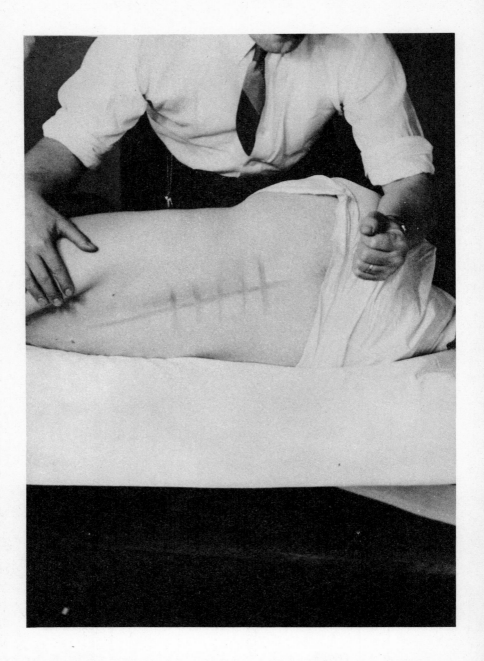

CONTINUING FORCE ON ISCHIAL TUBEROSITY CARRIES RO-
TATIONAL LOCKING UP TO INFERIOR OF THE TWO SEG-
MENTS.

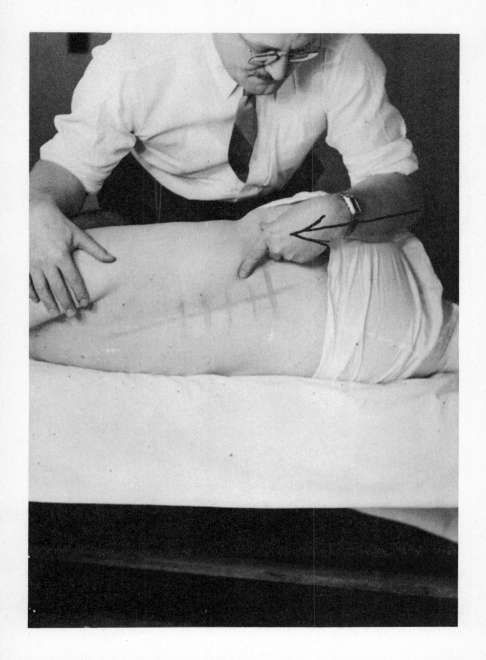

CORRECTIVE FORCE APPLIED BY CAUDAL ARM DIRECTING IT CEPHALWARD. DIRECT LATERAL FLEXIONED FORCE - NO ROTATION INVOLVED IN THE CORRECTIVE THRUST.

FLEXED LUMBAR FACET
PELVIC LIFT OR TWO MAN TECHNIQUE

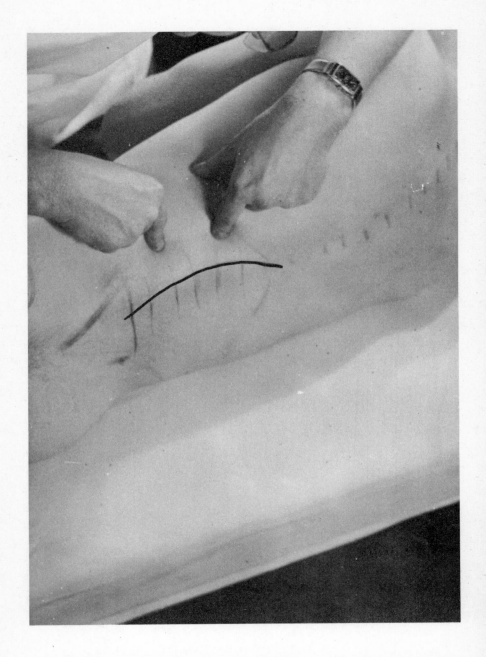

ILLUSTRATING THE CONVEX SIDE OR FLEXED FACET

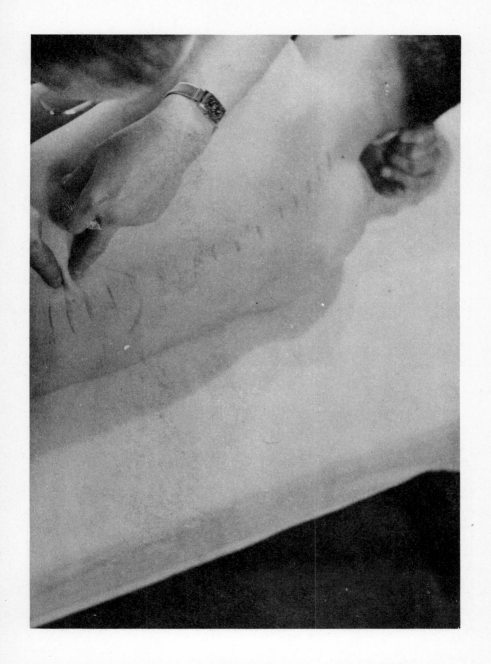

ILLUSTRATING THE EXTENDED FACET - THE OBJECTIVE OF
THE TECHNIQUE

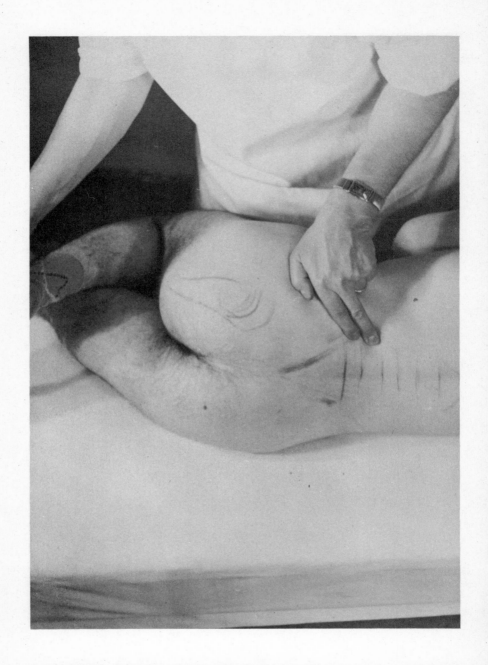

PATIENTS THIGHS ARE FLEXED ON PELVIS UNTIL MUSCLE TENSION ASCENDS TO THE LOWER OF THE TWO SEGMENTS IN LESION.

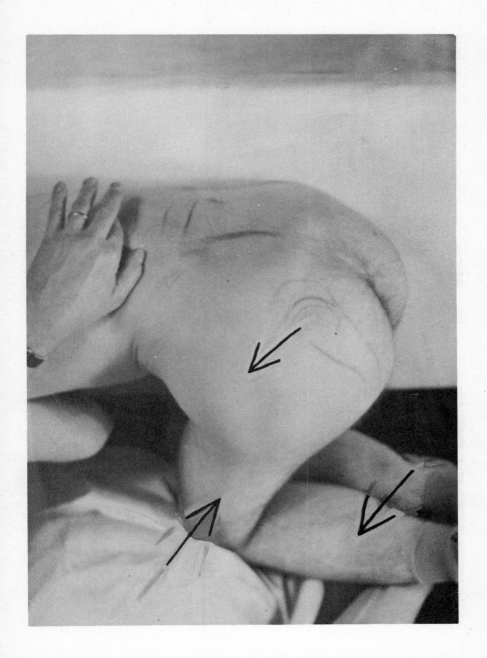

LEGS AND PELVIS ARE RAISED, KNEES DEPRESSED BY FORC-
ING PHYSICIAN'S THIGH AGAINST PATIENTS KNEE AND LOW-
ERING THEM. HAND UNDER LEGS, RAISED.

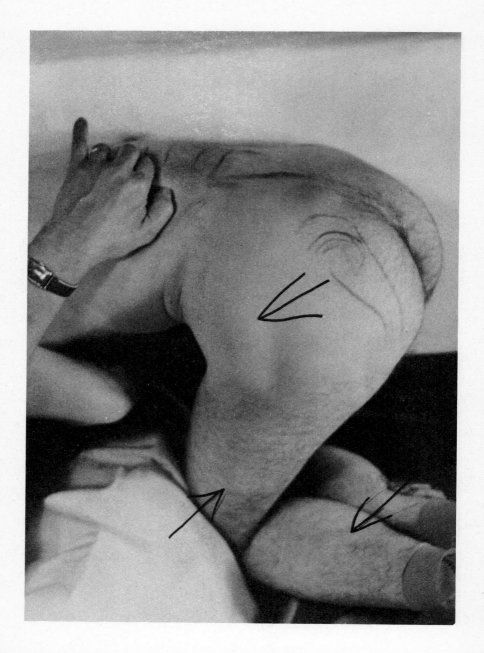

WHEN LATERAL FLEXION TENSION IS OBTAINED, A SHORT
THRUST IS TRANSMITTED BY THE PHYSICIAN-UPWARD ON
LEGS AND DOWNWARD ON KNEES OF PATIENT. THIS FORCES
THE PELVIS UPWARD AND CREATES A CONCAVITY ON EX-
TENDED FACET POSITION AT THE PALPATED LUMBAR LEV-
EL.

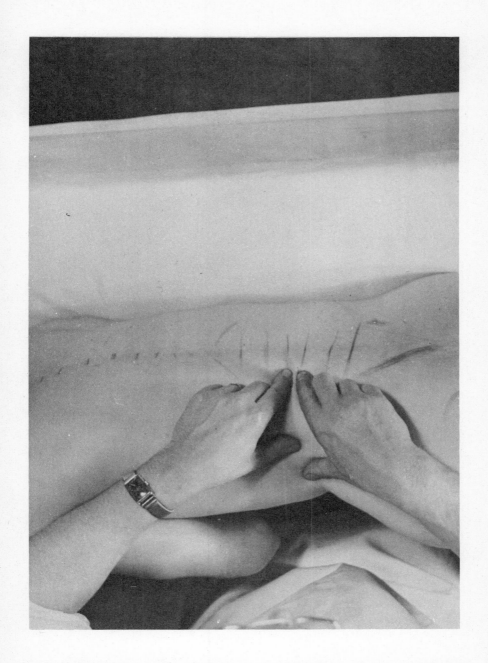

ILLUSTRATING THE CORRECTED LUMBAR AREA. FLEXED
FACETS NOW FORCED INTO EXTENDED POSITION.

FLEXED LUMBAR FACET
SITTING CORRECTION TECHNIQUE

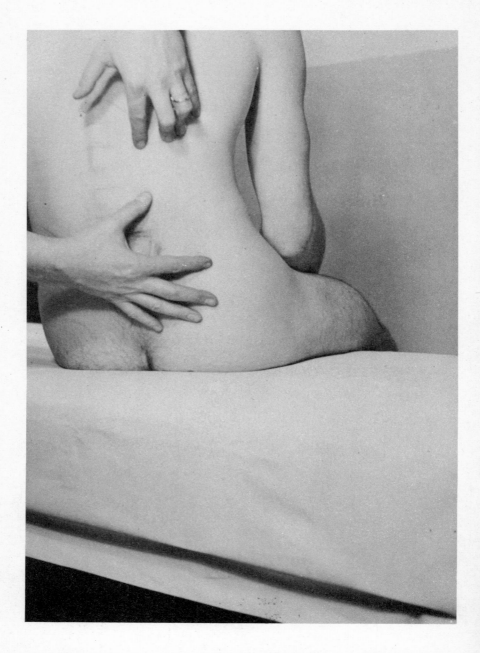

ILLUSTRATING SEPARATED TRANSVERSE PROCESSES ON FLEXED OR SEPARATED FACET SIDE ON THE CONVEXITY.

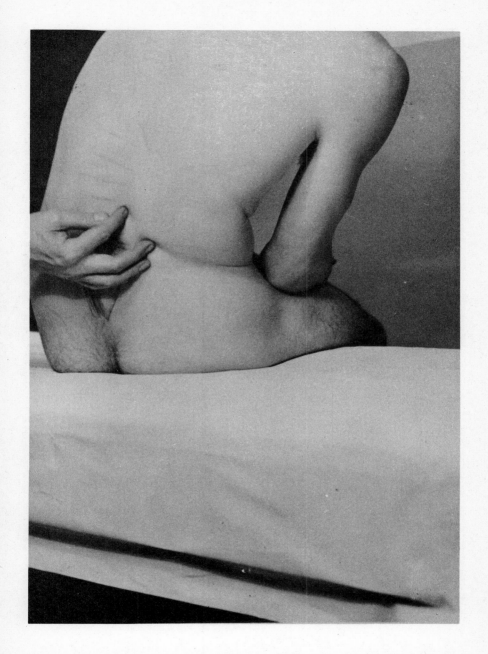

ILLUSTRATING THE APPROXIMATION OF THE ABOVE- THE
OBJECT OF TECHNIQUE TO ACQUIRE FULL RANGE OF MO-
TION.

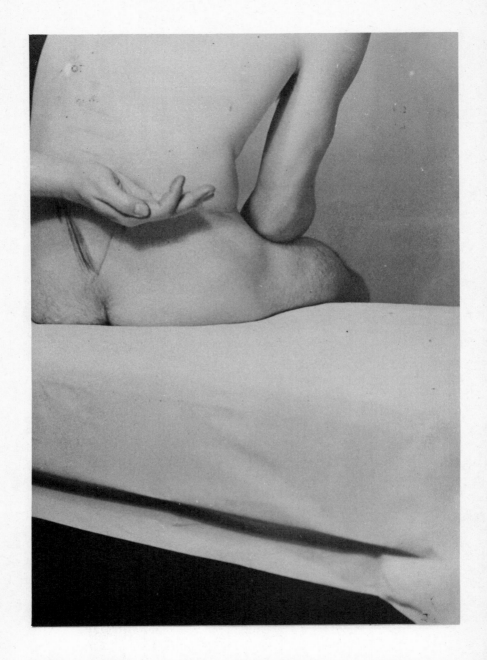

HYPOTHENAR EMINENCE FORCED UNDER THE TRANSVERSE
PROCESS OF THE INFERIOR OF THE TWO SEGMENTS.

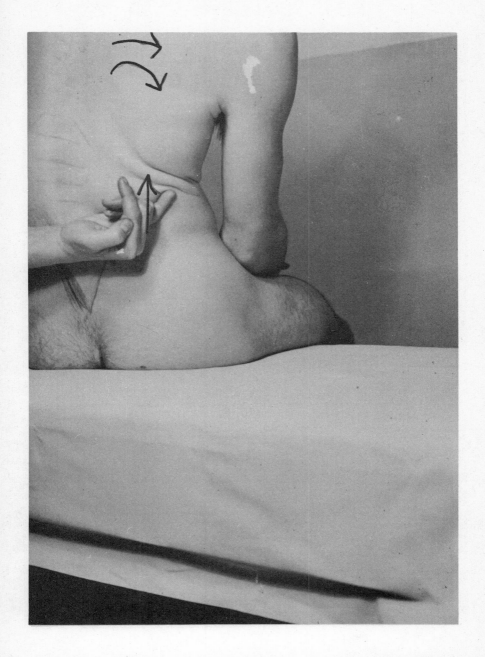

LATERAL FLEXION WITH ROTATION FROM ABOVE DOWN-
WARD TOWARD THE SIDE OF LESION, CARRYING THE ABOVE
SEGMENT DOWNWARD.

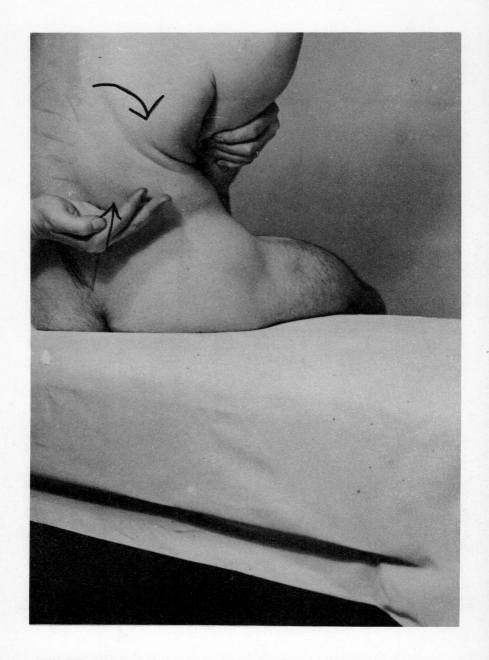

FORCE DIRECTED UPWARD ON THE INFERIOR SEGMENT AS
A CORRECTIVE AND COUNTER-FORCE.

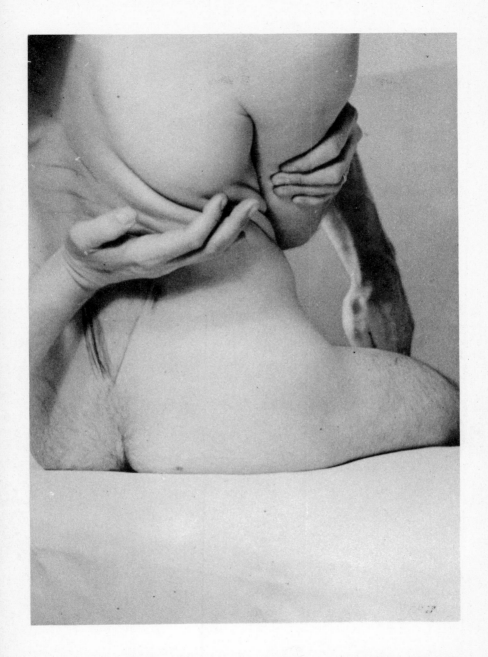

THRUST IS COMBINATION OF LATERAL FLEXION AND RO-
TATION FROM ABOVE AND A CEPHALIC LIFT.

EXTENDED LUMBAR FACET
LATERAL TECHNIQUE

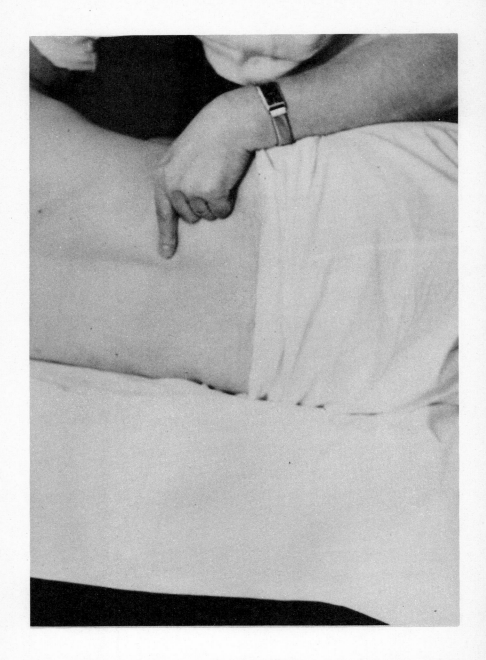

PALPATION OF THE RESTRICTED MOTION, MUSCLE SPASM, FIBROSIS, AND TRANSVERSE PROCESS APPROXIMATION ON THE SIDE OF THE EXTENDED FACET--ON THE SIDE TO WHICH SIDEBENDING AND ROTATION OF THE VERTEBRAL BODY OCCURS.

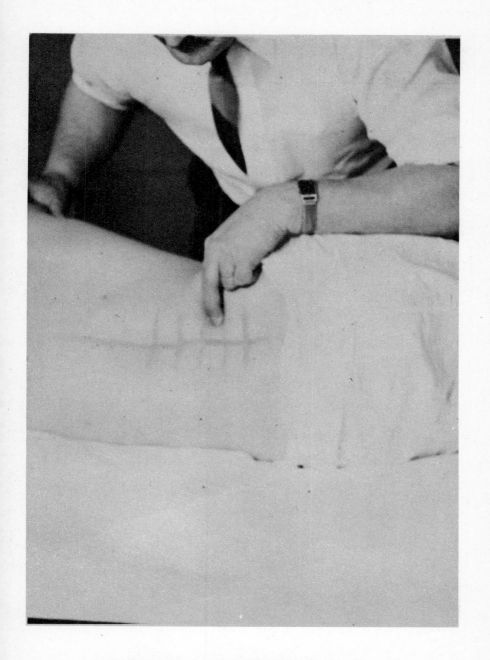

ILLUSTRATING THE EXTENDED FACET.

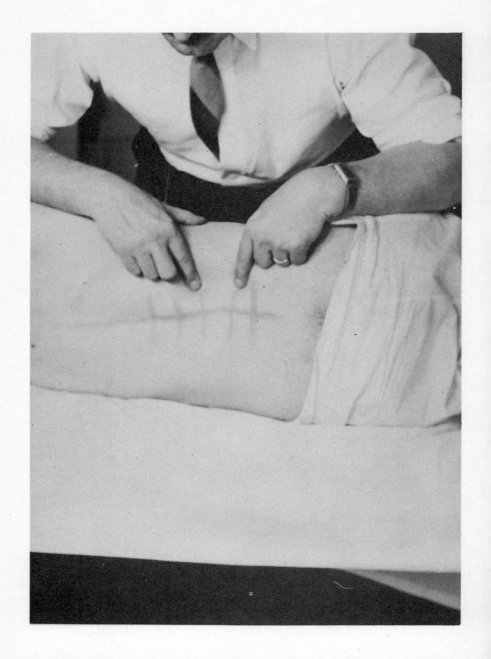

ILLUSTRATING THE DESIRED FLEXION OR SEPARATION OF
THE EXTENDED FACET--THE OBJECT OF THE TECHNIQUE.

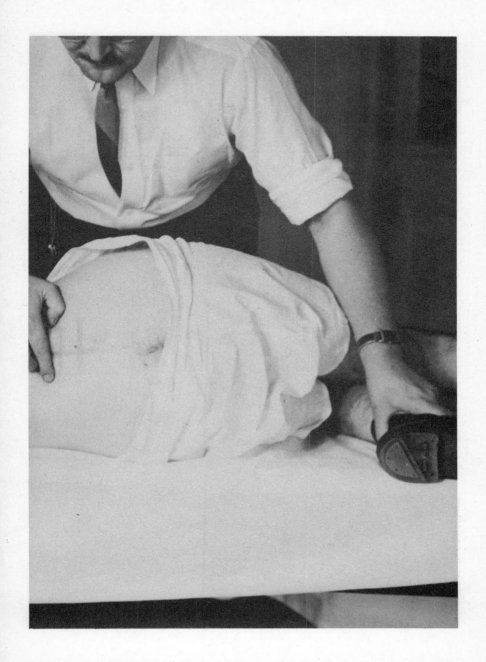

LOWER FEMUR IS FLEXED ON PELVIS UNTIL MUSCLE TEN-
SION ASCENDS TO THE INFERIOR OF THE TWO SEGMENTS.

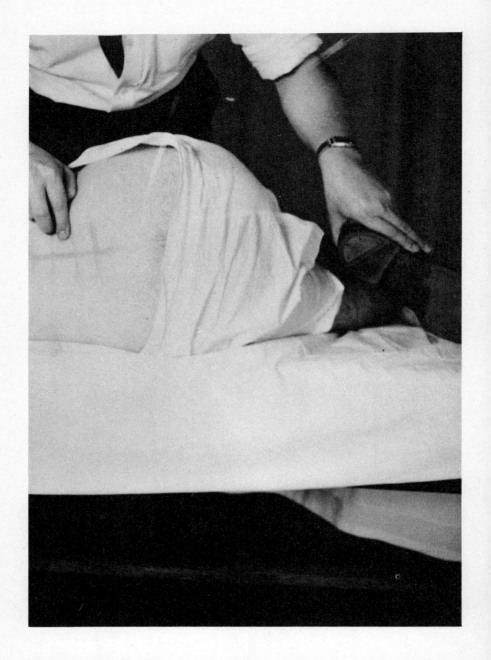

FOOT IS ANCHORED IN POPLITEAL SPACE SO LEG WILL NOT FALL OFF TABLE AND RESIST THE SUBSEQUENTLY APPLIED CAUDAL CORRECTIVE FORCE.

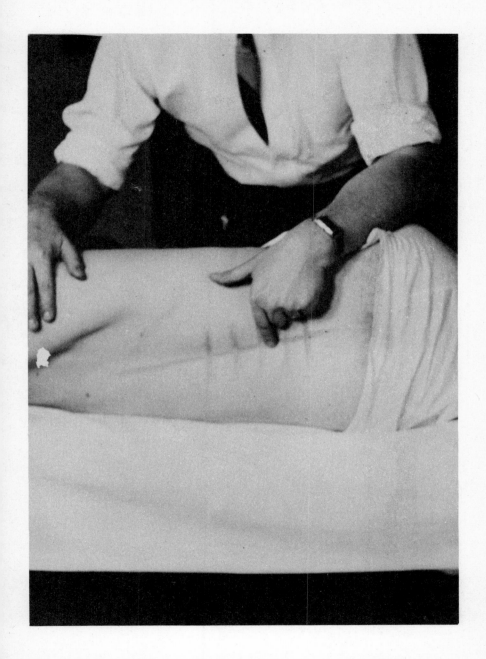

VERTEBRAL FACÉTS ARE PROTECTED BY TAKING OUT ALL
MOTION IN LATERAL FLEXION AND ROTATION DOWN TO THE
UPPER OF THE TWO SEGMENTS INVOLVED IN THE LESION.

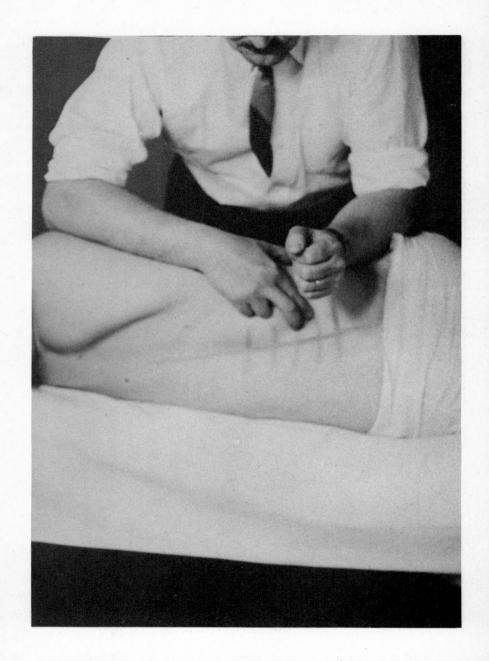

ILIUM IS BROUGHT ANTERIORLY AND INFERIORLY, AS ON A
FLEXED SACRUM, AND THE LUMBAR FACETS LOCKED IN
ROTATION UP TO THE INFERIOR OF THE TWO SEGMENTS.

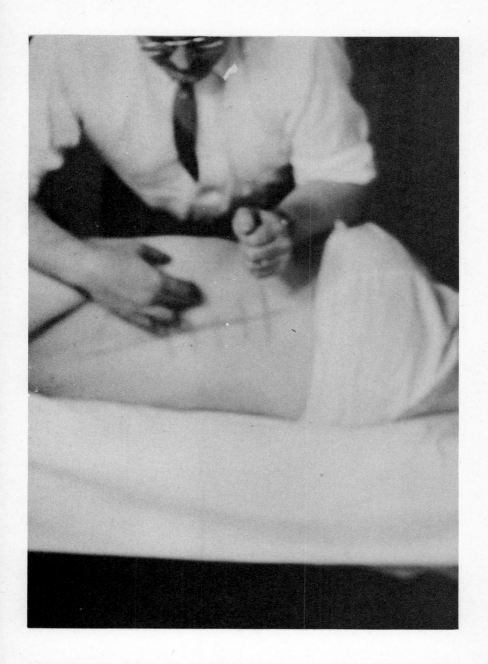

THIS LEAVES THE LESIONED ARTICULATION TO ASSUME THE
CORRECTIVE FORCE, THE ONES ABOVE AND BELOW BEING
PROTECTED. THE CORRECTIVE FORCE IS APPLIED ONTO THE
ILIUM AND LOCKED LUMBAR AREA FROM BELOW, PULLING
THE INFERIOR SEGMENT CAUDALLY FROM UNDER THE SU-
PERIOR ONE. THE CORRECTION IS OF HIGH VELOCITY AND
VERY LOW AMPLITUDE. FLEXION OR SEPARATION OF THE
EXTENDED OR OVERLAPPED FACET OCCURS.

EXTENDED LUMBAR FACET

SITTING TECHNIQUE

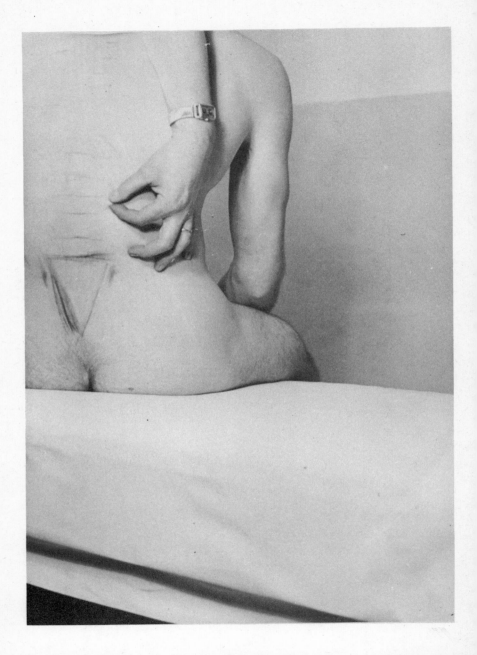

ILLUSTRATING THE TRANSVERSE PROCESS APPROXIMATION
ON THE EXTENDED FACET SIDE, OR THE CONCAVITY.

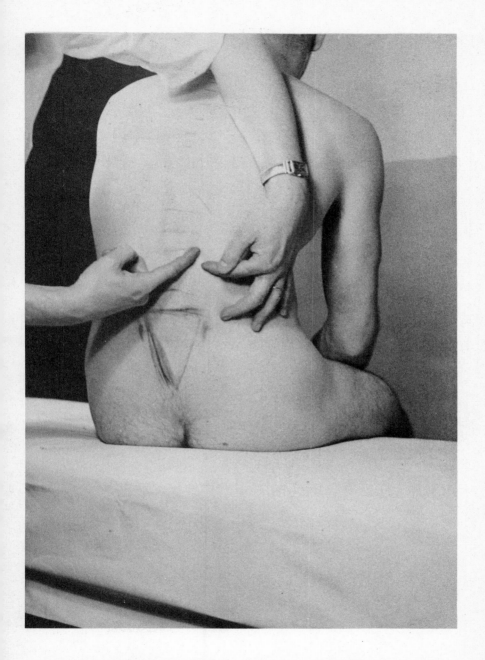

ILLUSTRATING THE OBJECTIVE OF THE TECHNIQUE—SEPARATION OR FLEXION OF THE EXTENDED FACET.

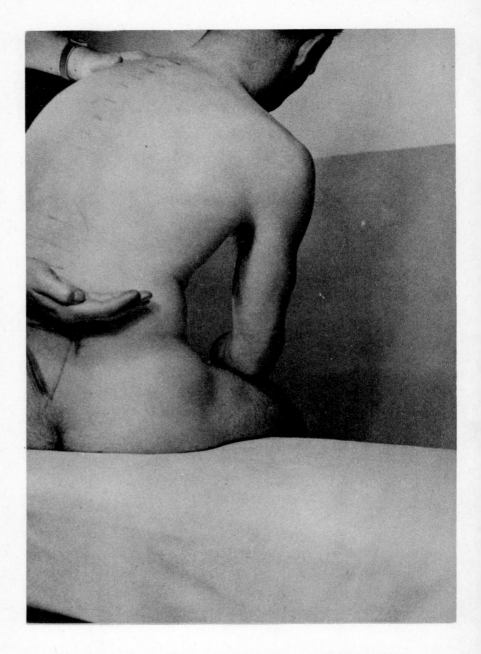

HYPOTHENAR EMINENCE IS FORCED BETWEEN THE TRANS-
VERSE PROCESSES COMPRESSING THE SOFT TISSUE.

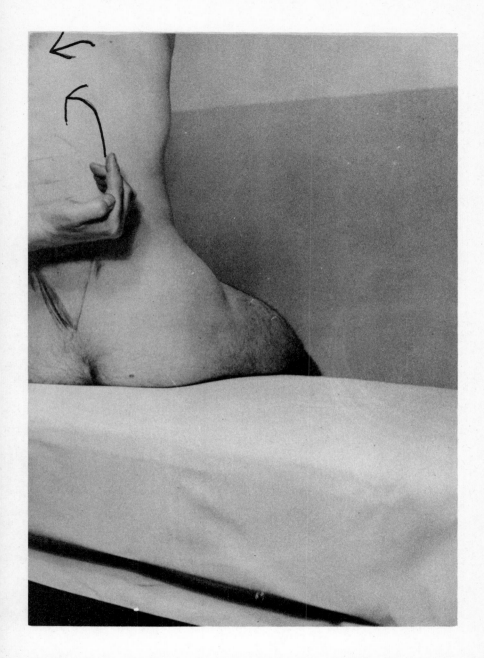

LATERAL FLEXION WITH ROTATION, PRODUCED BY OTHER ARM OVER SHOULDER, DOWN TO SEGMENT OF LESION.

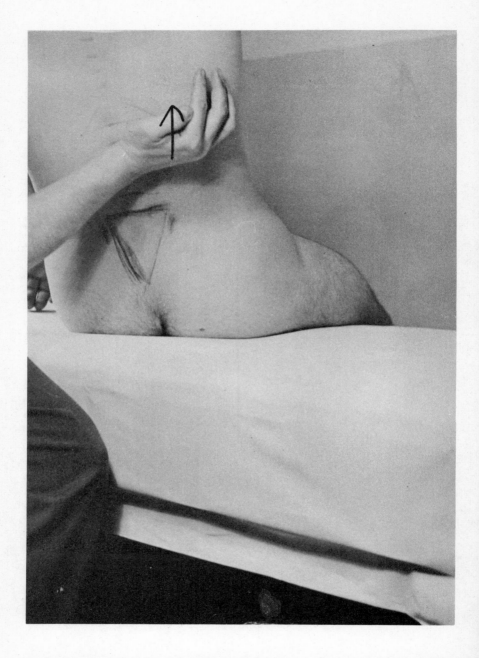

THRUST IS MADE BETWEEN TRANSVERSE PROCESSES, CAR-
RYING UPPER OF THE TWO SUPERIORLY FROM ITS EX-
TENDED POSITION INTO FLEXION.

THORACIC AREA

THORACIC AREA

The thoracic spinal area differs from the lumbar not so much in total range of motion, altho it is smaller, but in that the articular surfaces turn directly at right angles and face each other antero-posteriorly on a plane that travels laterally. The thoracic facet plane is directed from postero-inferior to supero-anterior at a forward angle of from 15 to 30°. There is resultantly considerable rotation combined with the lateral flexion phase, restricted progressively cephalward by the shorter and more intimately attached ribs.

Other peculiarities of the thoracic area include the change in direction of the normal curve. In the lumbar area it is lordotic; but at the dorso-lumbar juncture it changes, as do the facets in the opposite direction, and becomes kyphotic. This fact becomes doubly important in the biped. The kyphotic thoracic spine is increasingly susceptible to the detrimental force of gravity as aging develops, which it grieves me by 25 years or so to state, begins to exert its deliterious change at 20 to 25 years of age. Increase in the flexion state of the thoracic area intensifies the expirational position of the ribs and contributes its share toward embarrassed circulatory efficiency both to the viscera and to the spinal cord and lateral chain ganglia. This second phase would fill a book itself, but not a technique book. Therefore, this will have to be regretfully by-passed.

Normal respiration exerts interesting effects upon the thoracic cage. Upon inspiration there is a reduction of the flexional state. It does not go actually into the extended state but flexion is overcome by posterior inferior movement of the inferior facets of the vertebra above, upon the superior facets of the vertebra below. The transverse and spinous processes follow the facets, of course, which brings the rib angles downward and backward increasing the antero-posterior diameter of the thorax. Hence inspiration and rib leverage may be used adjunctively to move a flexed facet or expiratory rib lesion back into extensional or inspiratory position. The reverse associated motions of vertebra and rib occur in expiration, so expiratory muscle pull and rib leverage into expiratory position may be an aid to correction of an extended facet in the thoracic area or an inspiratory rib lesion.

Thoracic vertebral lesions may be held in the position of bilateral flexion, bilateral extension, or lateral flexion with rotation.

Rib lesions will be in inspiratory or expiratory position.

Inspiratory rib lesions are usually associated with an extended vertebral facet.

Expiratory rib lesions likewise are responsible for producing, or are the result of, usually, flexed vertebral facets. Trauma is of course etiological also.

Chart of the diagnostic points of thoracic vertebral and rib lesions will be found below.

Anatomical peculiarity necessitates further remarks relative to the thoracic area. The lower two ribs have no distal attachment; hence they can not be utilized as levers, and they should not receive specific thrusts. They will be pulled by muscle in superior or inferior position; consequently the musculature must receive treatment.

The upper two ribs are so densely bound to the vertbral transverse processes and the manubrium sterni that their independent mobility is slight. Being placed so high, the usual chest compression technique frequently becomes ineffective; hence the necessity of utilizing a cervical type of technique or typical upper dorsal technique.

BILATERAL THORACIC LESIONS

	BILATERAL EXTENSION	BILATERAL FLEXION
Body of vertebra above on one below	Moved postero-inferiorly	Moved antero-inferiorly
Spinous process	Approximates one below. Motion restricted in area of approximation.	Approximates one above. Motion restricted in area of separation.
Transverse process	Postero-inferior. Approximates one below. Prominent.	Antero-superior. Approximates one above. Less prominent.
Rib	Carried postero-inf. into inspiratory state	Carried antero-superiorly into expiratory state.

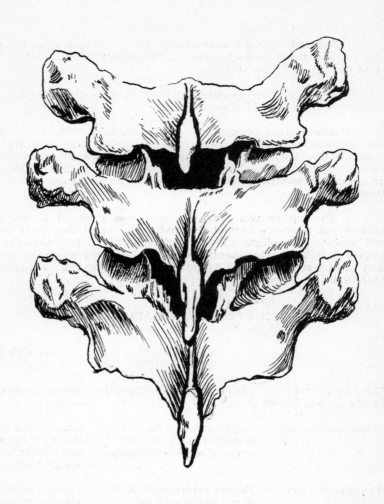

BILATERAL FLEXION

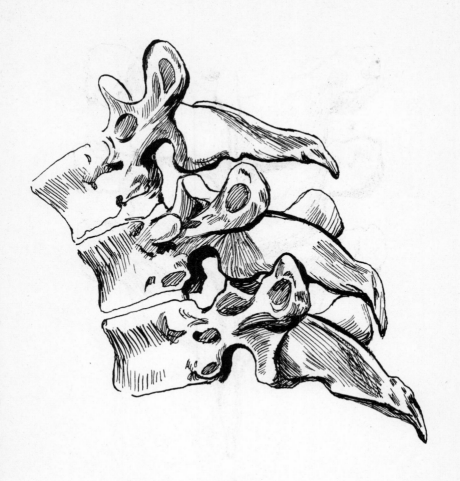

BILATERAL FLEXION

LATERAL VIEW

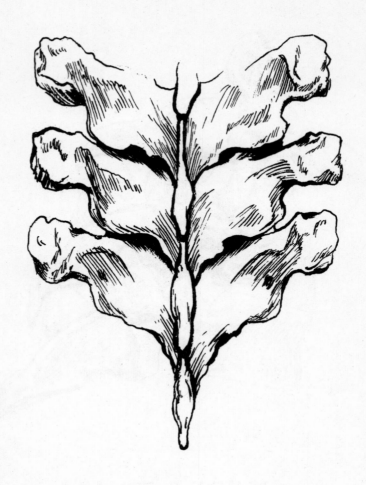

BILATERAL EXTENSION

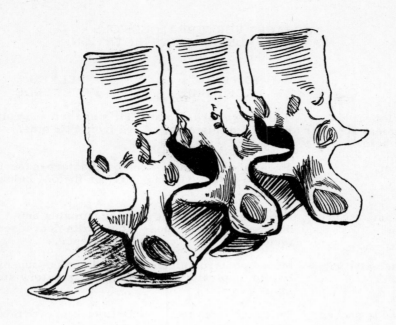

BILATERAL EXTENSION

LATERAL VIEW

THORACIC VERTEBRAL LESIONS -
LATERAL FLEXION WITH ROTATION

	EXTENDED FACET SIDE	FLEXED FACET SIDE
Vertebral body of segment above on one below	Tilts downward. Rotated toward this side.	Tilts upward and rotated from this side.
Facet	Facet above moved postero-inferiorly on one below.	Moved antero-superiorly on the one below.
Transverse process	Approximates the one below. Prominent posteriorly.	Approximates one above with decreased prominence.
Associated rib	Moved postero-inferiorly into inspiratory state	Moved antero-superiorly into expiratory state.
Spinous process	Deflected from this side	Deflected toward flexed facet side.

RIB LESIONS

	INSPIRATORY	EXPIRATORY
Rib angle	Postero-inferior. Prominent. Approximates one below	Antero-superior. Less prominent. Approximates to one above.
Inferior border	Less prominent	More prominent
Front of rib	More prominent	Less prominent
A-P diameter of rib	Increased. More horizontal.	Lessened. Decreased more horizontal.

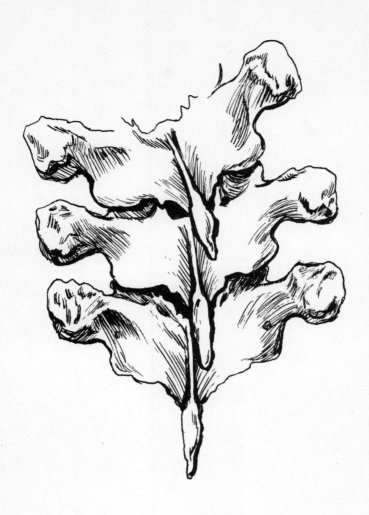

LATERAL FLEXION

WITH ROTATION

BILATERAL FLEXION LESIONS
CHEST COMPRESSION RIB LEVERAGE TECHNIC

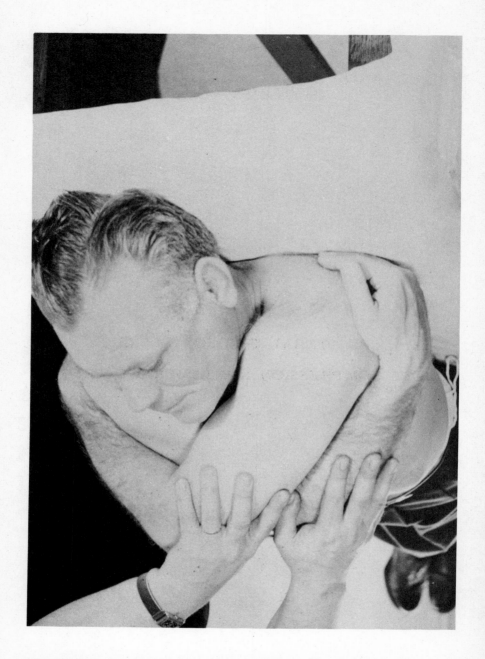

TECHNIQUE FOR BILATERAL FLEXION OF VERTEBRAL FAC-
ETS WITH OR WITHOUT BILATERAL EXPIRATORY RIBS. IL-
LUSTRATING POSITION OF ARMS TO PRODUCE RIB LEVERAGE.

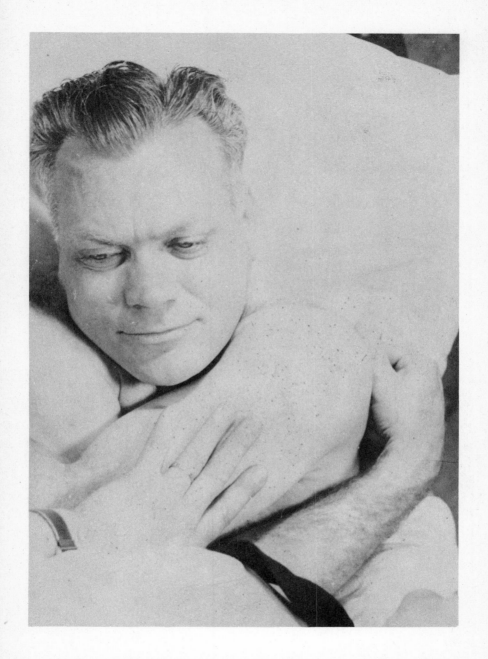

PATIENT'S FURTHER ARM IS PLACED ON TOP OF THE CLOS-
ER ARM.

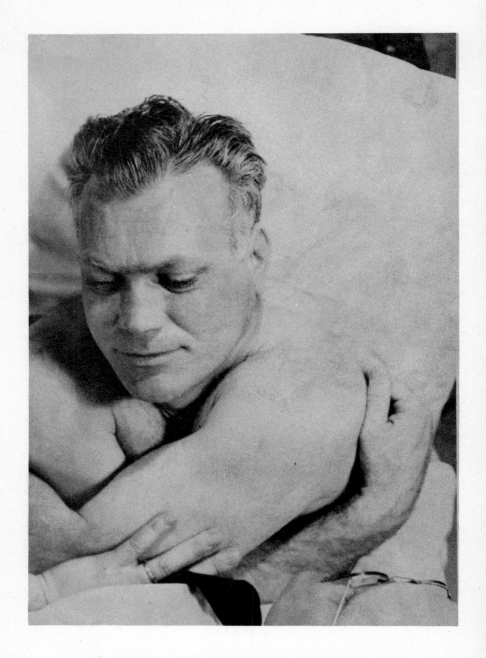

PATIENT IS ROTATED TOWARD PHYSICIAN.

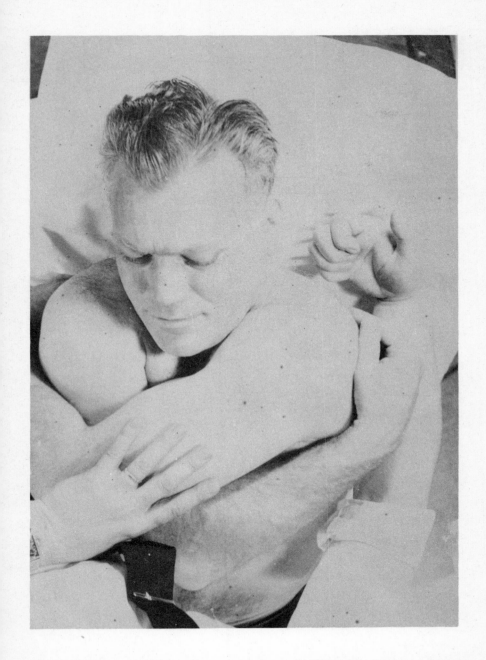

POSITION OF CORRECTIVE HAND - METACARPO-PHALANGEAL
ARTICULATIONS STRAIGHT. PHALANGES FLEXED. SPINOUS
PROCESSES WILL FALL IN THE CONCAVITY.

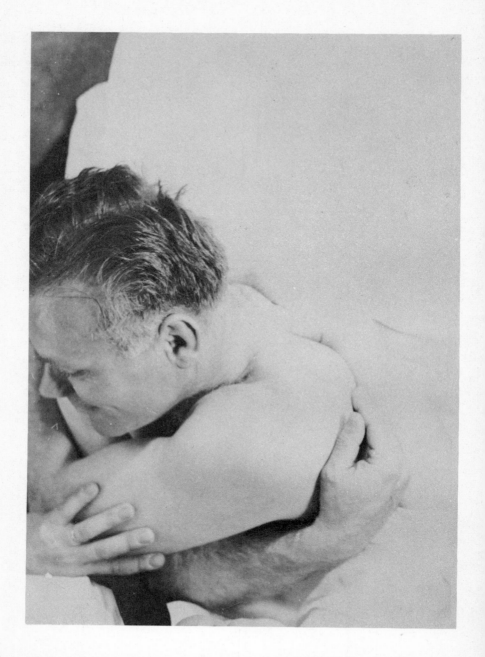

HAND IN POSITION. THENAR AND HYPOTHENAR EMINENCES CONTACTING TRANSVERSE PROCESSES AND RIBS ON ONE SIDE, FLEXED FINGERS ON THE OTHER.

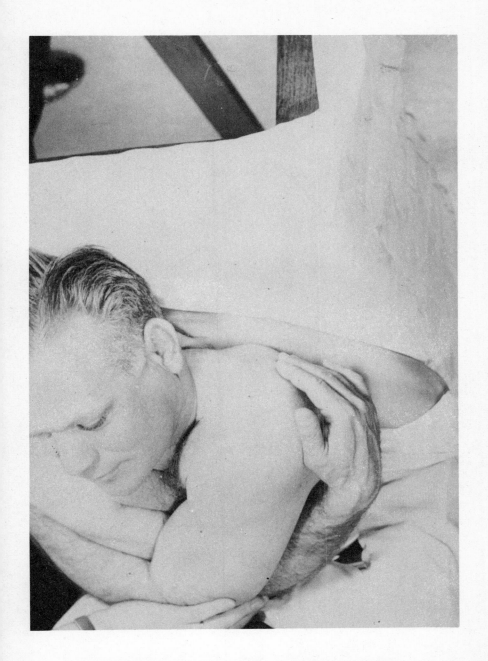

PATIENT ROLLED ONTO CORRECTIVE HAND.

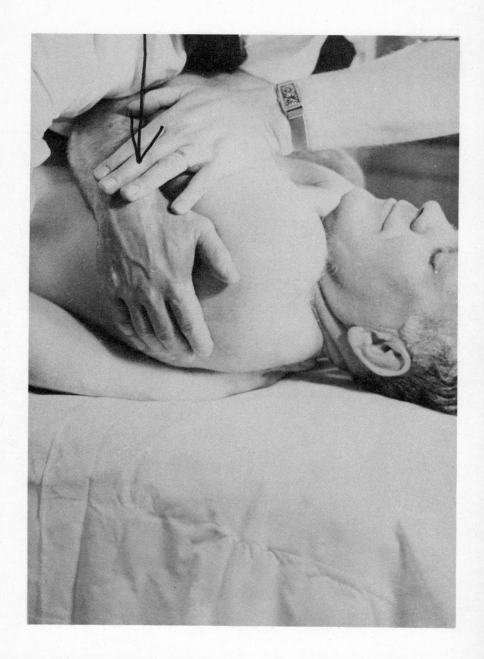

IN THE EXPIRATORY PHASE 25 to 50 POUNDS IS PLACED ON
THE HAND COVERING THE PATIENT'S ELBOWS, AND TRANS-
MITS THAT WEIGHT TO THE RIBS.

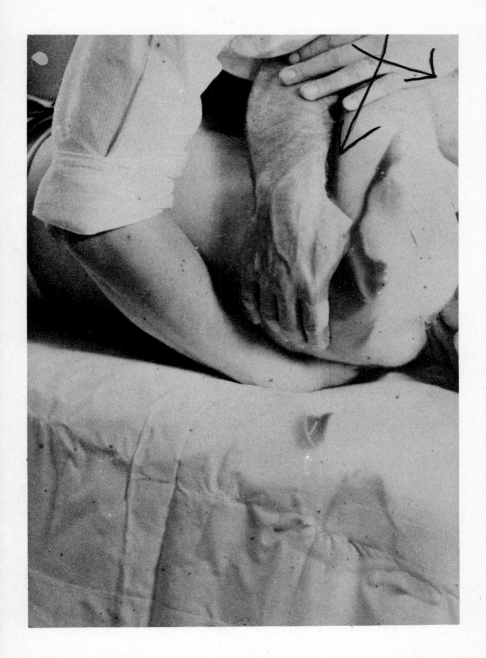

PATIENT INHALES FORCEFULLY; RIBS ARE RAISED INTO IN-
SPIRATORY POSITION; RIB LEVERAGE AGAINST HAND FORCES
VERTEBRAL FACETS TO EXTEND UPON EACH OTHER.
THRUST IS RARELY NEEDED.

FLEXED THORACIC FACET - EXPIRATORY RIB
UNILATERAL TECHNIQUE

FLEXED THORACIC FACET

The flexed or "anterior" facet has moved antero-superiorly with relation to the facet of the vertebra below. Vertebral body rotates to the opposite side and tilts to the opposite side.

The transverse process of the vertebra below must be fixed with the thenar eminence to prevent its moving as we attempt to force the facet and rib above into extension and inspiratory position.

The thenar musculature should be contracted. The hand should be flat and positioned cross-wise of the back under the rib and transverse process of the vertebra below.

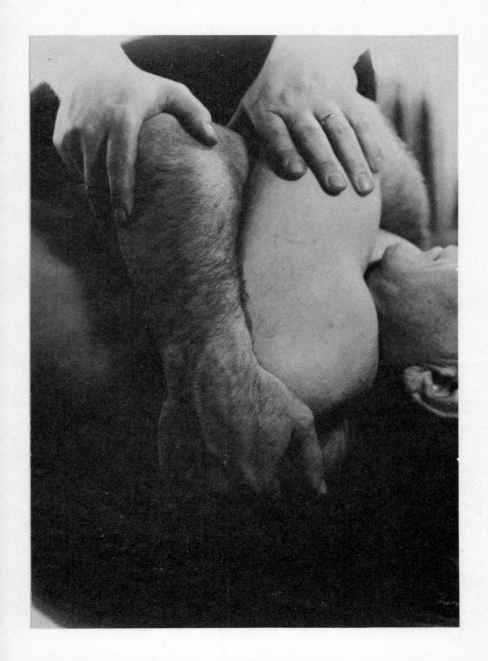

POSITIONING OF ARMS OVER THE FRONT OF THE RIB OF INVOLVED FACET.

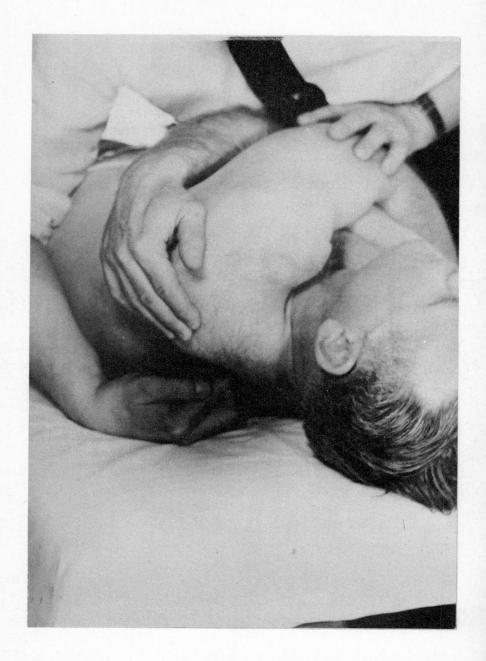

ILLUSTRATING THE TRANSVERSE PROCESS OR RIB ANGLE OF
THE VERTEBRA BELOW. THENAR EMINENCE IS PLACED UN-
DER THESE TO FORCE THEM UP UNDER THE ABOVE.

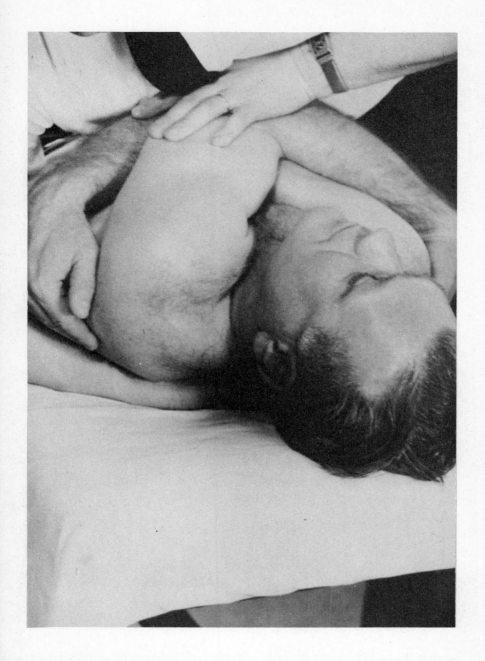

FORCED EXPIRATION PLACES ALL RIBS IN EXPIRATORY PO-
SITION AND FACETS INTO FLEXION. 25 TO 50 POUNDS IS
APPLIED ON FRONT OF RIB.

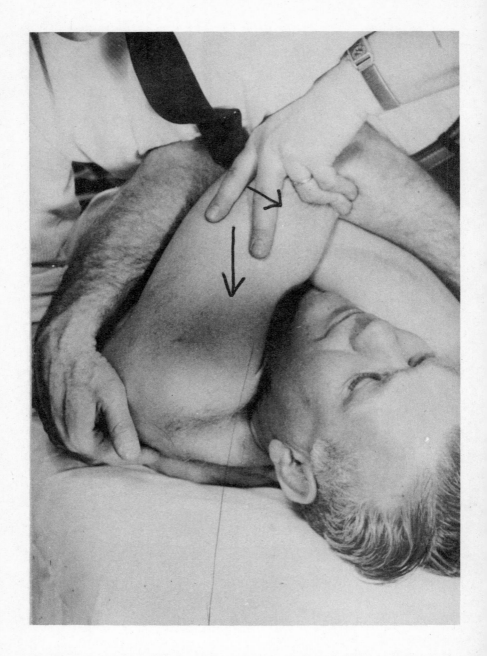

FORCED EXPIRATION AND WEIGHT ROLLING UP OVER THE
THENAR EMINENCE FORCES RIB INTO INSPIRATORY POSI-
TION AND FLEXED FACET INTO EXTENSION POSITION.

UPPER DORSAL FLEXED FACET
AND ELEVATED RIB TECHNIQUE

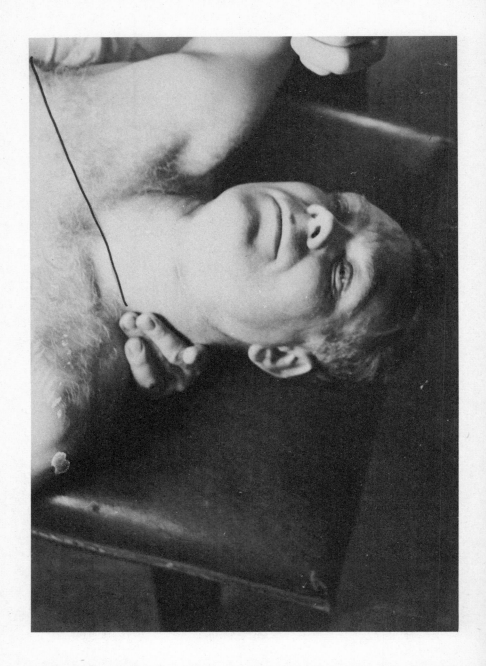

RECOMMENDED TECHNIQUE FOR ELEVATED RIB AND/OR
FLEXED VERTEBRAL FACET AT 1st or 2nd THORACIC LEVEL.
CAUDAL HAND PASSES UNDER PATIENT, AXILLA- BODY AND
MIDDLE FINGER LIES ALONG THE RIB TO ITS ANTERIOR END.

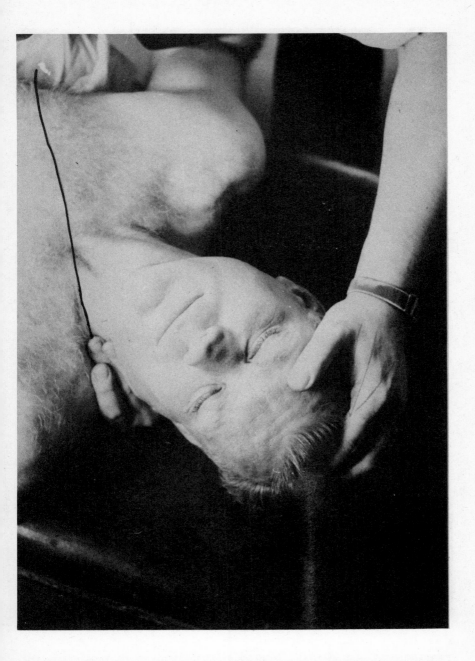

CEPHALIC HAND LATERALLY FLEXES AND ROTATES IF POSSIBLE TOWARD THE CORRECTIVE HAND PRODUCING COUNTERFORCE.

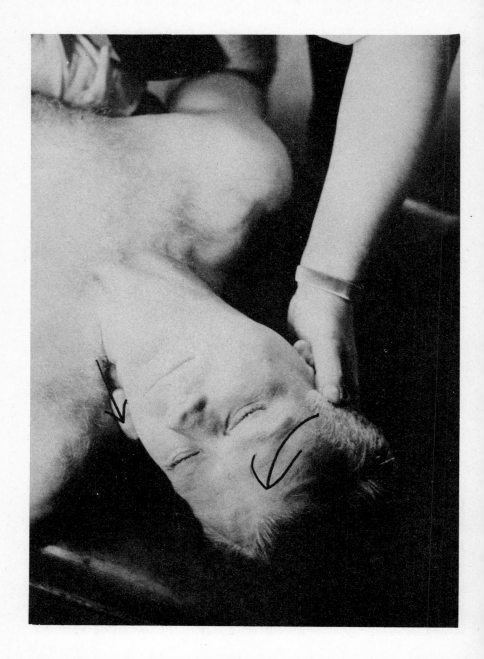

TENSION IS SECURED. CORRECTIVE FORCE IS APPLIED BY
THE HAND ON RIB, CARRYING IT POSTERO-INFERIORLY MOV-
ING IT DOWNWARD AND THE VERTEBRAL FACET INTO EX-
TENSION FROM ITS PREVIOUSLY FLEXED POSITION. THE
WHOLE SEGMENT IS DE-ROTATED.

RIB LEVERAGE FLEXED FACET TECHNIQUE

PATIENT SITTING

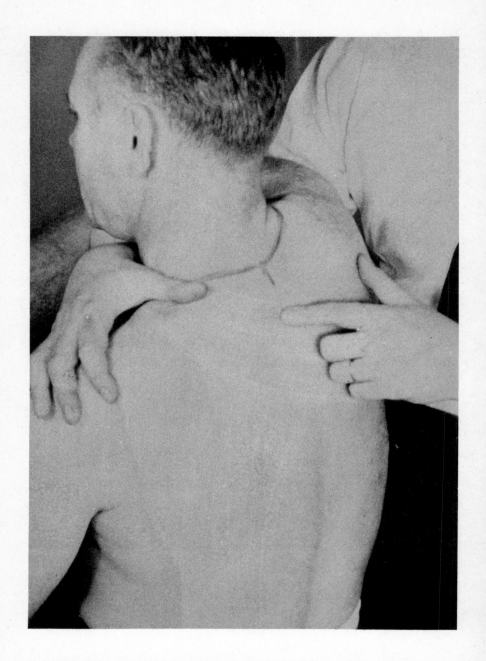

A LESS DESIRABLE SITTING TECHNIQUE. VENTRAL HAND PLACED WITH THUMB OVERLYING ELEVATED RIB. THUMB POINTING IN DIRECTION RIB AND VERTEBRA IS TO BE MOVED. APPROACH IS UNDER OPPOSITE AXILLA. PATIENT'S ARM OVER PHYSICIAN'S SHOULDER.

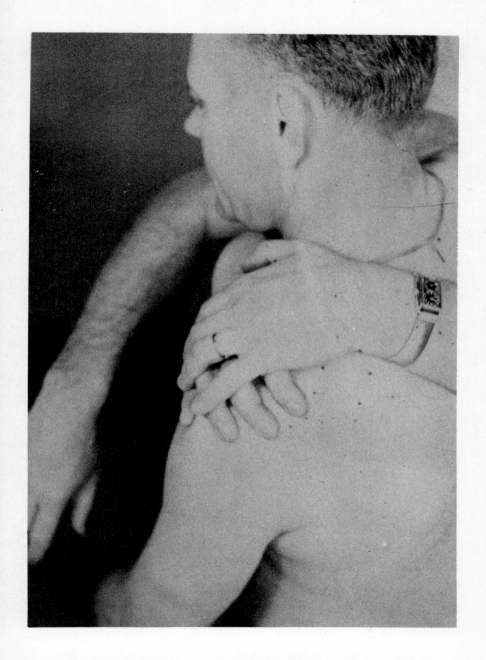

CORRECTIVE HAND RE-INFORCED BY OTHER HAND.

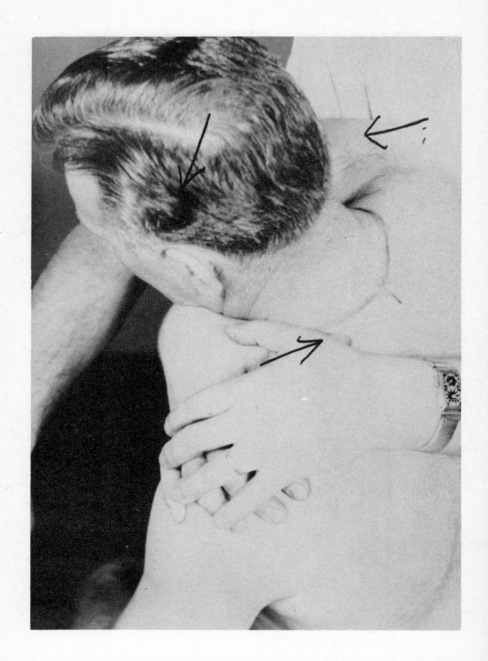

PATIENT'S OPPOSITE ARM IS RAISED AND CORRECTIVE HAND
PULLS POSTERO-INFERIORLY ON THE ELEVATED RIB. PA-
TIENT IS SIDE BENT TOWARD LESIONED SIDE WHICH AIDS
THE RIB DESCENT, FACET EXTENSION, AND DE-ROTATION OF
VERTEBRA.

FLEXED FACET ELEVATED RIB TECHNIQUE
PATIENT SITTING

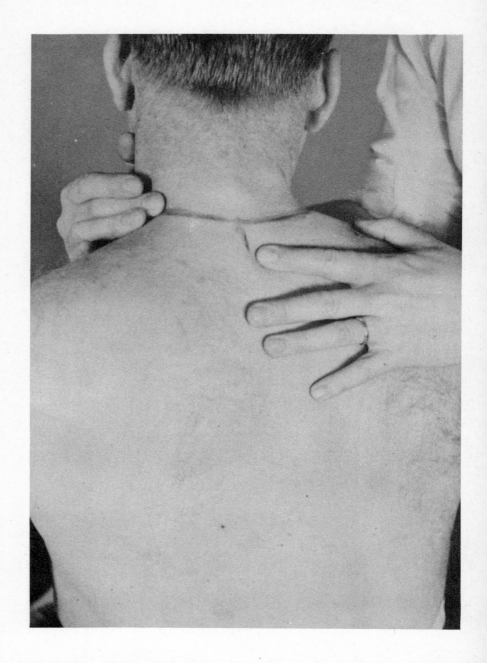

ILLUSTRATING POSITION OF LATERAL FLEXION AND ROTA-TION. SPINOUS PROCESS DEVIATED TO SIDE ON WHICH TRANSVERSE PROCESS AND RIB HAVE MOVED ANTERO-SU-PERIORLY--PROMINENT THEREFORE ABOVE. ON THE OP-POSITE OR EXTENDED FACET SIDE, THE FACET AND RIB HAVE MOVED POSTERO-INFERIORLY.

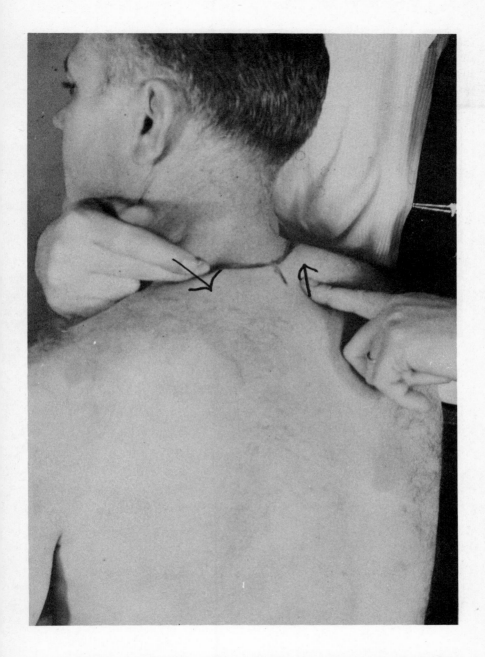

ILLUSTRATING REVERSAL MOTION, THE OBJECTIVE OF TECHNIQUE. ELEVATED RIB, FLEXED FACET SIDE, MAY BE USED AS LEVER.

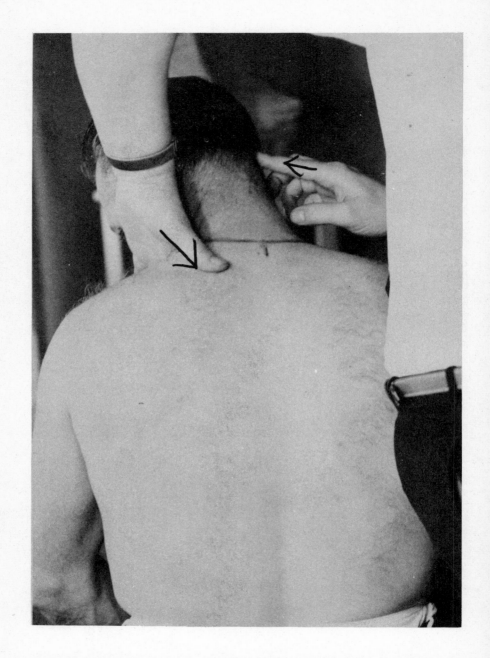

CORRECTIVE HAND ON FRONT AND SUPERIOR ASPECT OF
RIB. HEAD LATERALLY FLEXED AND ROTATED TO SAME
SIDE TO AID IN EXTENDING FLEXED FACET AND RELAXING
ANTERIOR SCALENUS MUSCLE.

322

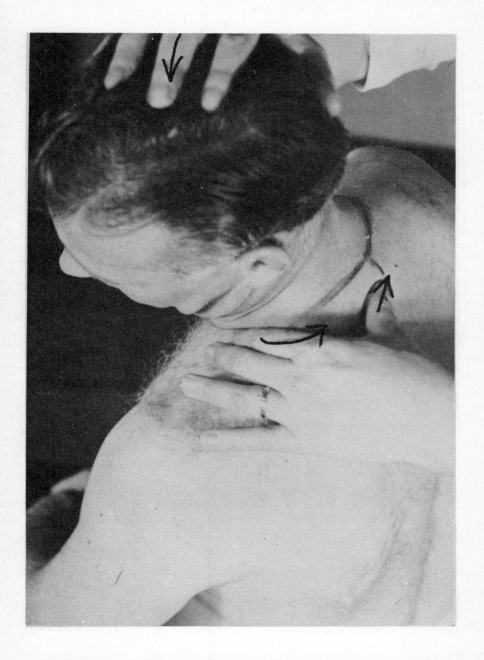

CORRECTIVE THRUST CARRIES ELEVATED RIB AND/OR
FLEXED FACET POSTERO-INFERIORLY TO NORMAL POSITION.
ADDITIONAL THRUST MAY BE GIVEN BY THUMB ON SIDE OF
SPINOUS PROCESS AIDING THE DE-ROTATION.

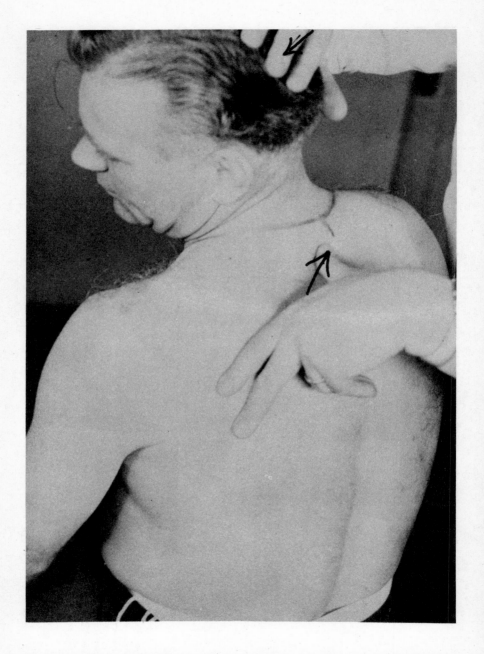

SIMILAR TECHNIQUE-USING SPINOUS PROCESS CORRECTION ALONE.

FLEXED FACET - ELEVATED RIB
CERVICAL TYPE TECHNIQUE

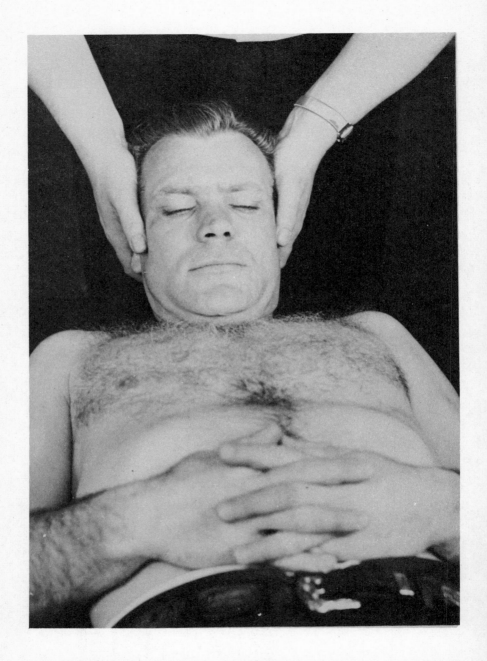

SUPINE PATIENT, CERVICAL TECHNIQUE FOR SAME CORREC-
TION. HEAD POSITIONED NORMALLY.

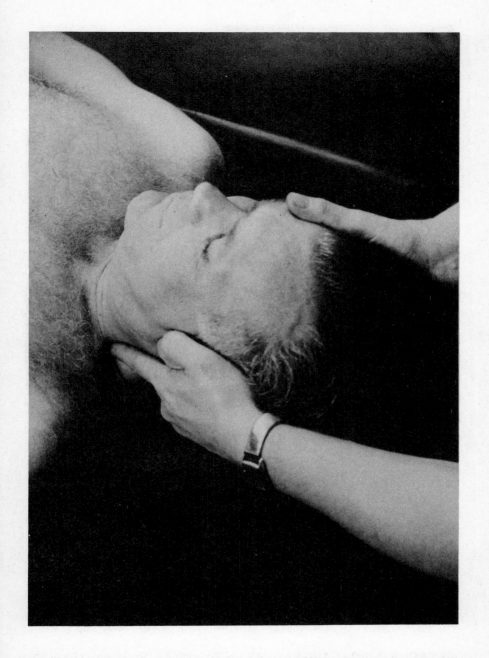

FINGER CONTACTS ANTERO-SUPERIOR ASPECT OF ELEVATED
RIB, FLEXED FACET SIDE.

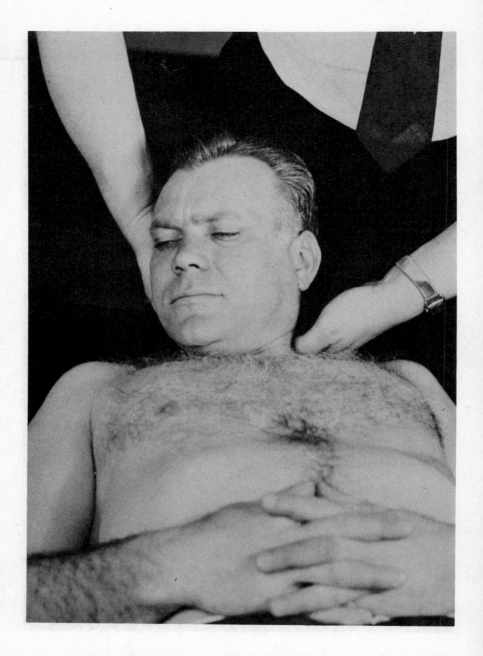

METACARPOPHALANGEAL ARTICULATION PLACED IN POSITION FOR CORRECTIVE THRUST.

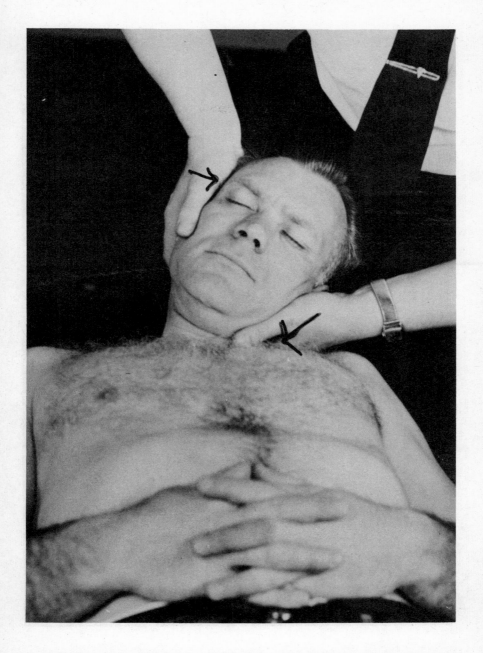

OTHER HAND LATERALLY FLEXES AND ROTATES HEAD AND
CERVICAL SPINE OVER CORRECTIVE HAND FOR COUNTER-
FORCE AND TO RELAX ANTERIOR SCALENUS MUSCLE.

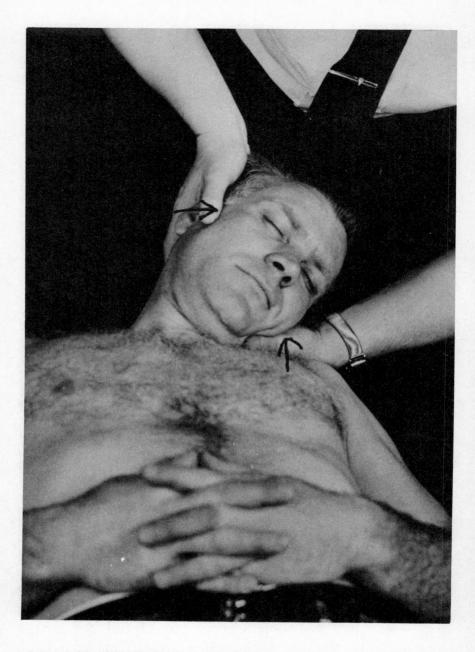

CORRECTIVE THRUST ON RIB-CARRYING IT POSTERIOR-IN-FERIORLY, EXTENDING THE FLEXED FACET AND DEROTAT-ING THE VERTEBRA.

FLEXED FACET - ELEVATED RIB SPINOUS PROCESS TECHNIQUE

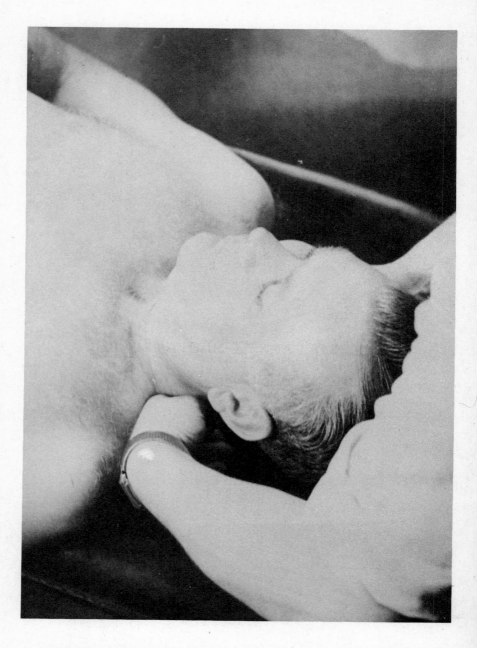

CERVICAL APPROACH - TO SPINOUS PROCESS TECHNIQUE
IN UPPER DORSAL AREA, APPLICABLE FROM 1ST TO 5TH
OR 6TH THORACIC AND UPPER DORSAL CURVATURE, CAR-
DIAC CURVE, "CARDIAC SAG".

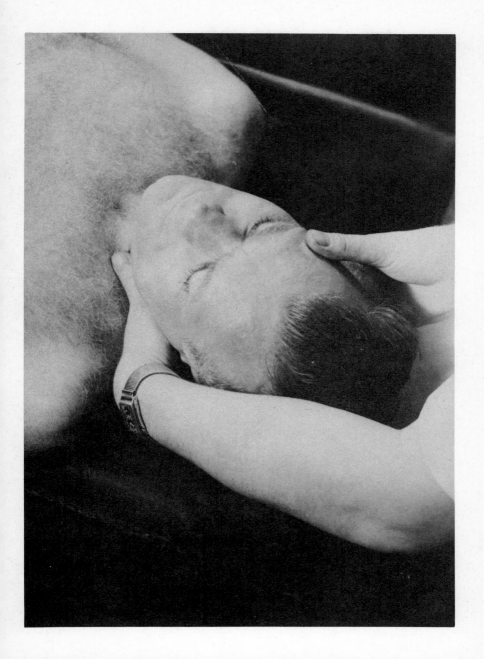

CORRECTIVE HAND ON SIDE OF SPINOUS PROCESS ON FLEXED
FACET, ELEVATED OR EXPIRATORY RIB SIDE.

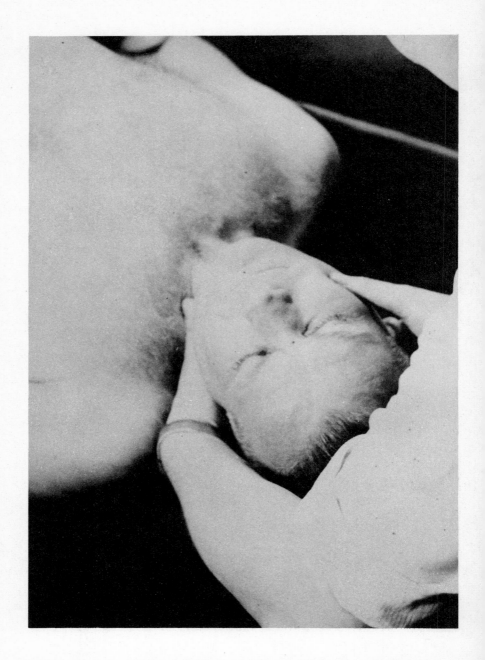

CEPHALIC HAND LATERALLY FLEXES AND ROTATES HEAD
AND CERVICAL SPINE TOWARD CORRECTIVE HAND, RELAX-
ING SCALENI AND PROTECTING CERVICAL FACETS.
CORRECTIVE HAND THRUSTS POSTERO-INFERIORLY, ON FULL
INSPIRATION, DEPRESSING RIB, EXTENDING FACET AND DE-
ROTATING VERTEBRA.

FLEXED FACET - LOWER THORACIC AREA
PATIENT SITTING

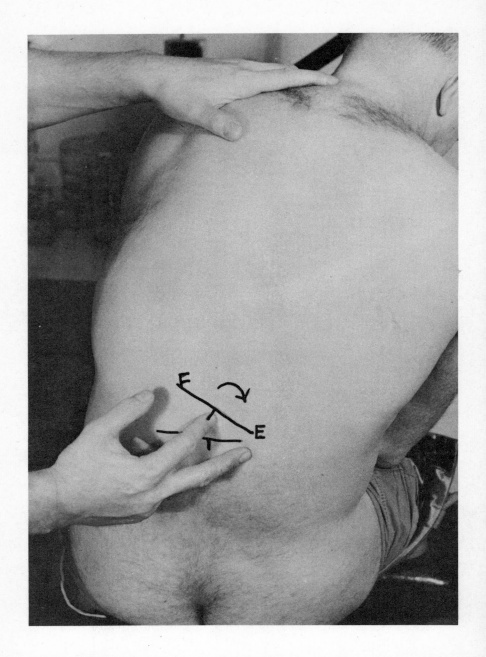

FLEXED FACET TECHNIQUE: PATIENT SITTING. ILLUSTRAT-
ING THE GROSS LATERAL FLEXION WITH ROTATION TO THE
CONCAVITY. SEPARATED FACETS AND TRANSVERSE PROC-
ESSES ON THE CONVEXITY.

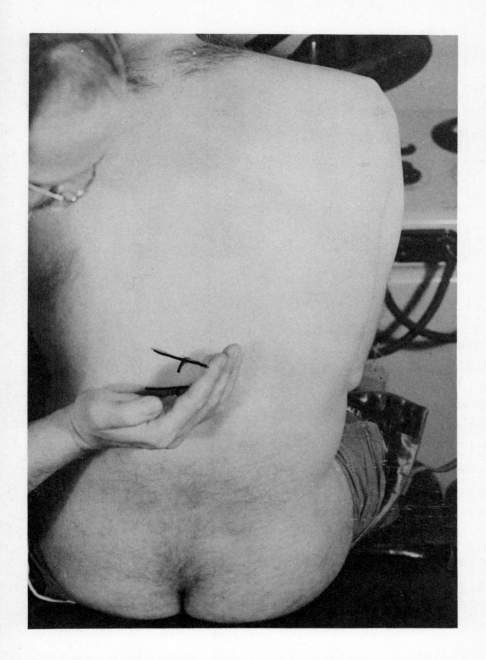

HYPOTHENAR EMINENCE FORCED UNDER THE TRANSVERSE PROCESS BELOW. PATIENT LATERALLY FLEXED AND ROTATED TOWARD FLEXED FACET IN CORRECTIVE DIRECTION.

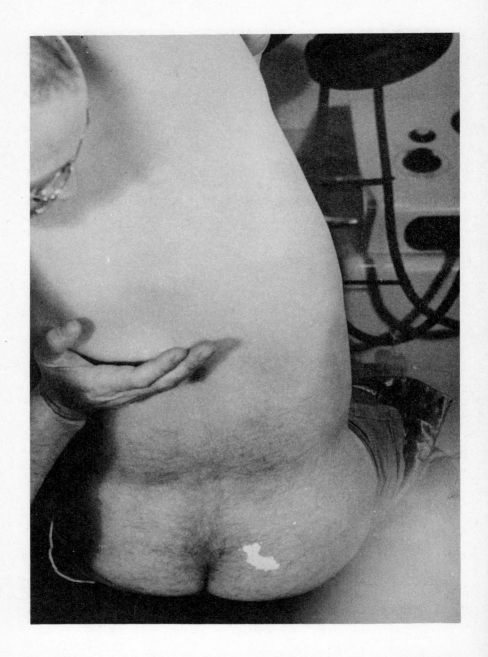

THRUST IS EXERTED UNDER THE INFERIOR TRANSVERSE
PROCESS, CARRYING IT SUPERIORLY UNDER THE ONE ABOVE.

EXTENDED FACET - INSPIRATORY RIB
RIB LEVERAGE TECHNIQUE WITH
CHEST COMPRESSION

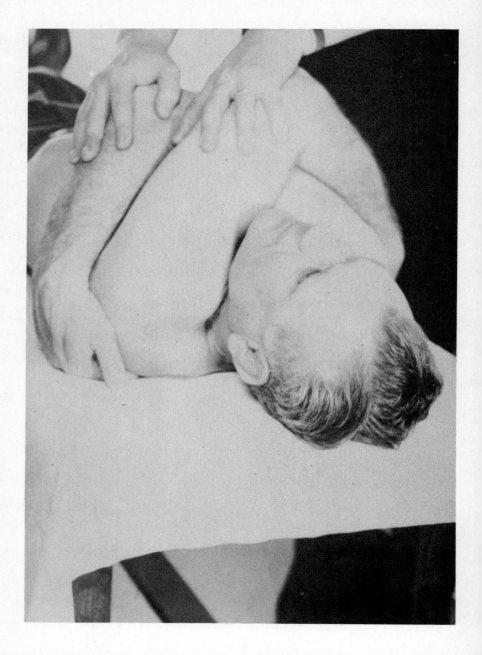

POSITIONING OF PATIENTS ARMS FOR EXTENDED FACET OR
INSPIRATORY RIB LESION CORRECTION.

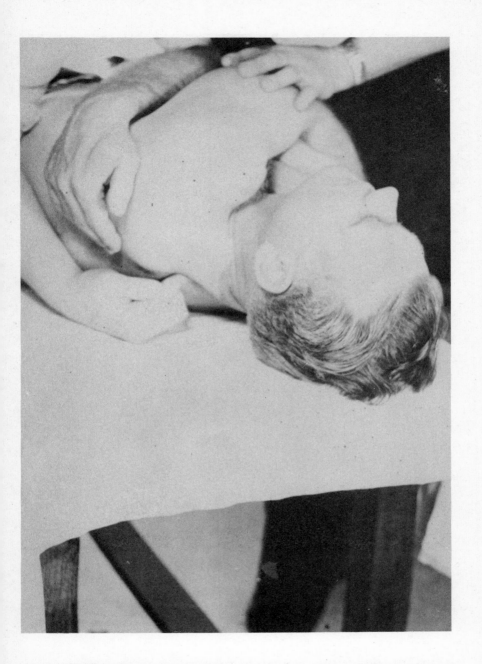

PALPATING THE POSITION FOR THE CORRECTIVE HAND.

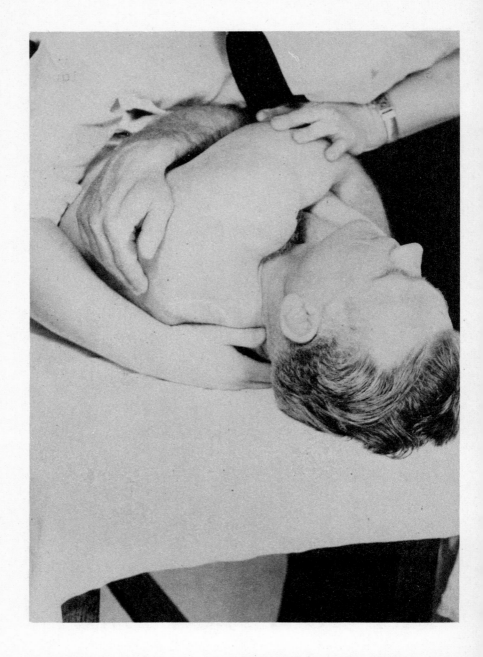

HAND IN POSITION – THENAR EMINENCE UNDER EXTENDED
TRANSVERSE PROCESS ON ANGLE OF INSPIRATORY RIB.

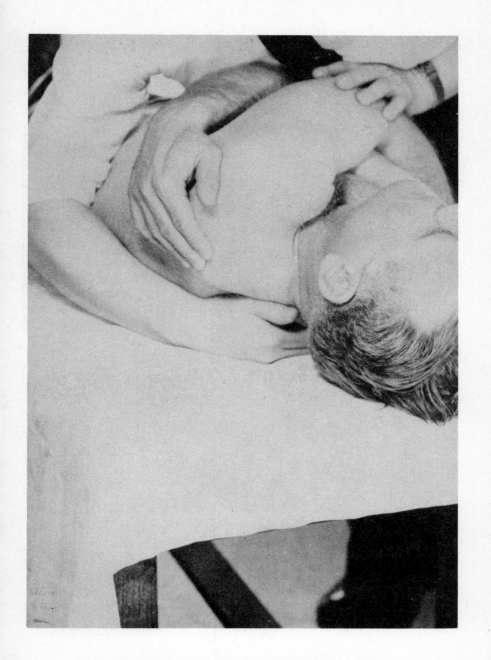

PATIENT IS ROLLED EASILY ONTO BACK.

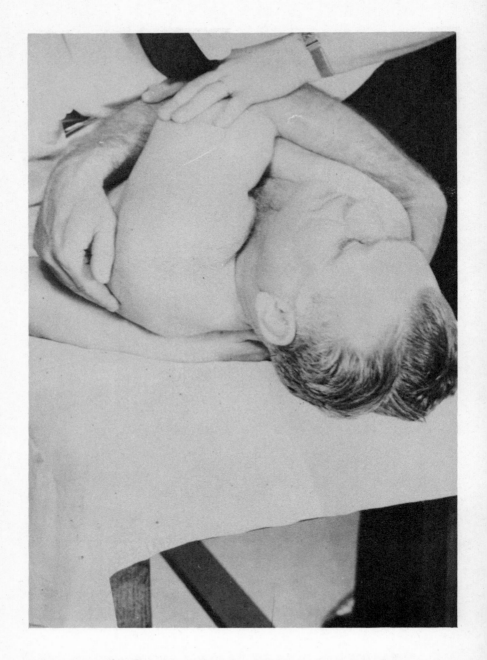

CARE IS TAKEN TO MAKE CERTAIN OF THENAR CONTACT,
REMAINING HAND IS FLAT.

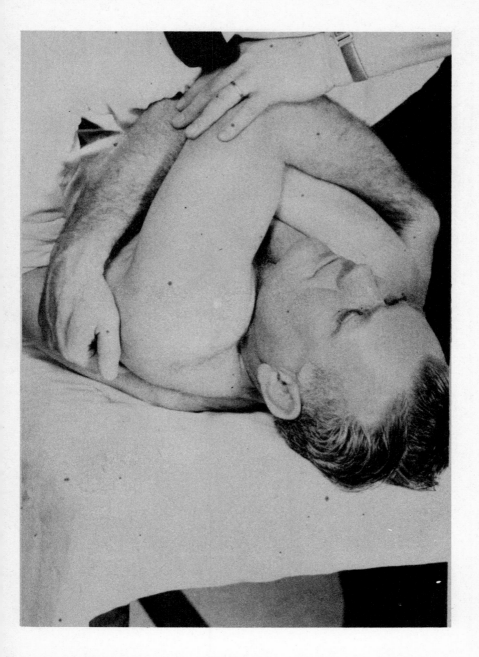

ON FULL BREATH, WEIGHT (25 TO 50 LBS.) IS PLACED ON
HAND OVER PATIENT'S ELBOWS, TRANSMITTING THIS WEIGHT
TO RIBS.

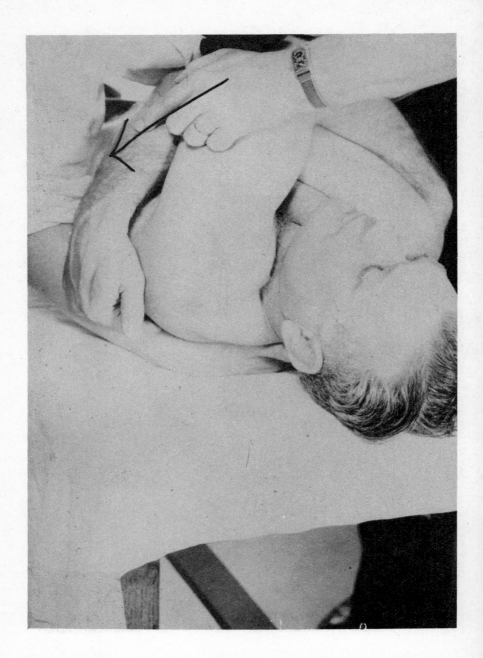

PATIENT FORCEFULLY EXHALES. WEIGHT RIDES FRONT OF
RIBS DOWN INTO EXPIRATORY POSITION. WEIGHT AND EX-
PIRATORY EFFORT FORCES TRANSVERSE PROCESS AND RIB
AGAINST THENAR EMINENCE WHICH FORCES TRANSVERSE
PROCESS INTO FLEXED POSITION AND RIB INTO EXPIRA-
TORY STATE. THRUST IS RARELY NEEDED.

EXTENDED FACET

INSPIRATORY RIB - UPPER DORSAL AREA

CERVICAL TYPE TECHNIQUE

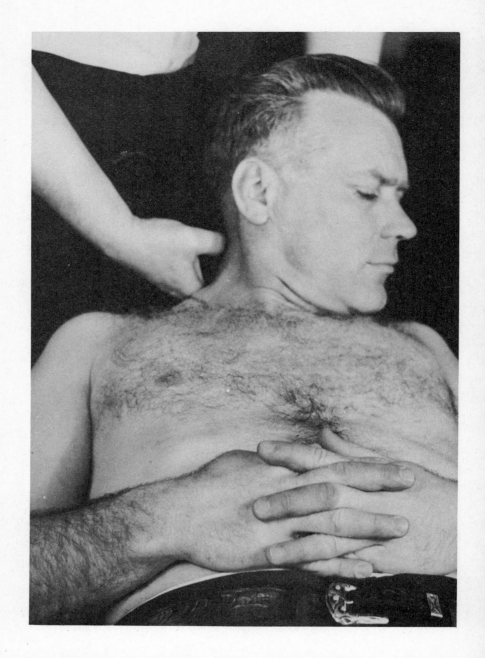

MODIFIED CERVICAL TECHNIQUE MAY BE USED FOR THE EXTENDED VERTEBRAL FACET ON INSPIRATORY RIB IN UPPER DORSAL AREA. CORRECTIVE HAND (METACARPO-PHALANGEAL ARTICULATION OF INDEX FINGER) APPLIED UNDER TRANSVERSE PROCESS AND/OR RIB.

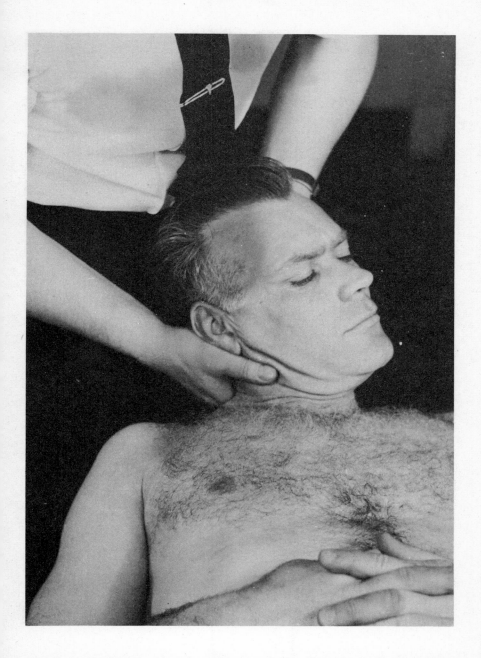

COUNTERFORCE PRODUCED BY LATERALLY FLEXING CERV-
ICAL SPINE ONLY, JUST DOWN TO THE CORRECTIVE HAND.
NO LOWER.

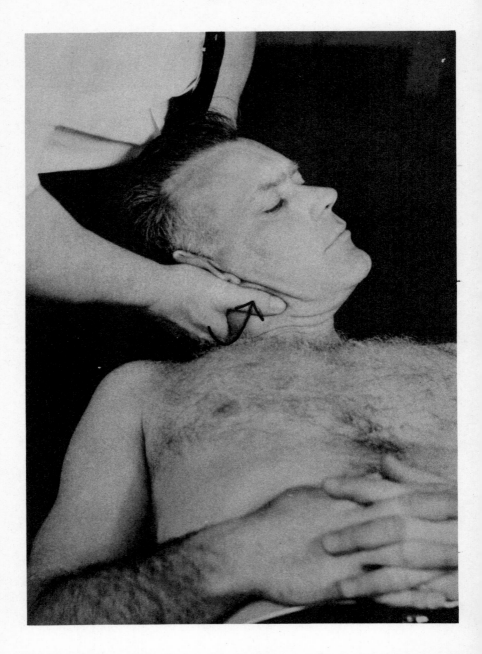

CORRECTIVE HAND CARRIES ARTICULAR FACET TRANSVERSE PROCESS AND RIB ANTERO-SUPERIORLY, PARALLEL WITH ARTICULAR SURFACE; TENSION IS ACCUMULATED MILDLY, SUDDEN, SHORT, SHARP, CORRECTIVE LIFT APPLIED TO CORRECTIVE HAND. HAND HOLDING HEAD IS PASSIVE, ONLY MAINTAINING COUNTERFORCE.

EXTENDED FACET - INSPIRATORY RIB
TRANSVERSE PROCESS TECHNIQUE

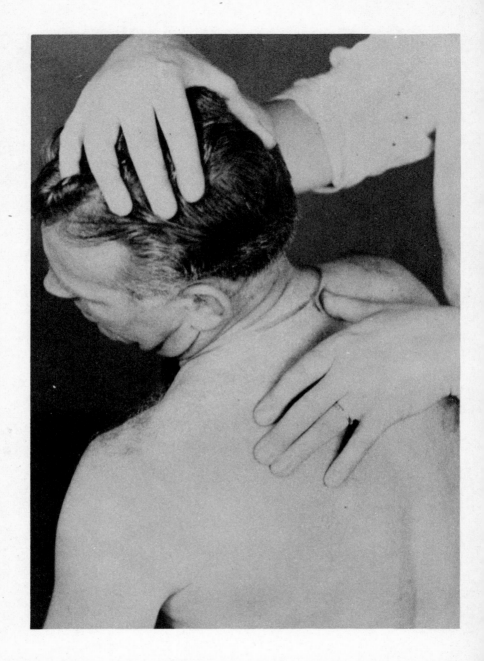

EXTENDED TRANSVERSE PROCESS CORRECTION. THUMB PLACED UNDER THE TRANSVERSE PROCESS AND DEPRESSED RIB. HEAD LATERALLY FLEXED STRONGLY TO OPPOSITE SIDE TO IMITATE FACET FLEXION AND TO PULL ANTERO-SUPERIORLY ON DEPRESSED RIB.

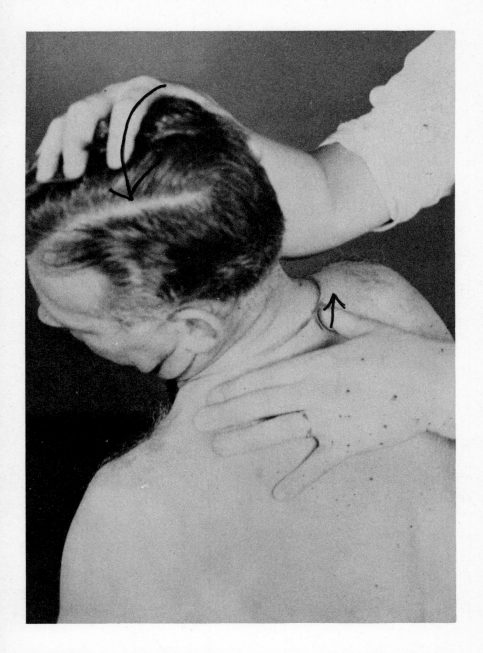

TENSION SECURED, THRUST IS MADE ANTERO-SUPERIORLY
UNDER THE TRANSVERSE PROCESS AND RIB, DE-ROTATING
VERTEBRA.

EXTENDED FACET - INSPIRATORY RIB

KNEE - TRANSVERSE PROCESS TECHNIQUE

PATIENT SITTING

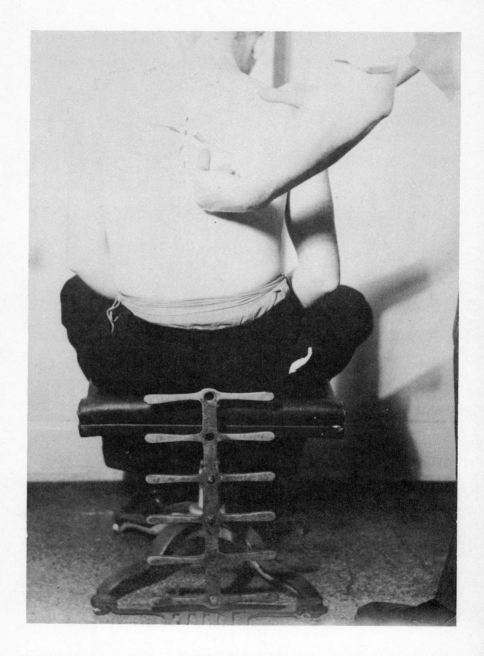

KNEE TECHNIQUE APPLIED TO EXTENDED TRANSVERSE
PROCESS. ILLUSTRATING DIRECTION OF LIFT NECESSARY
TO SEPARATE THE APPROXIMATED FACETS.

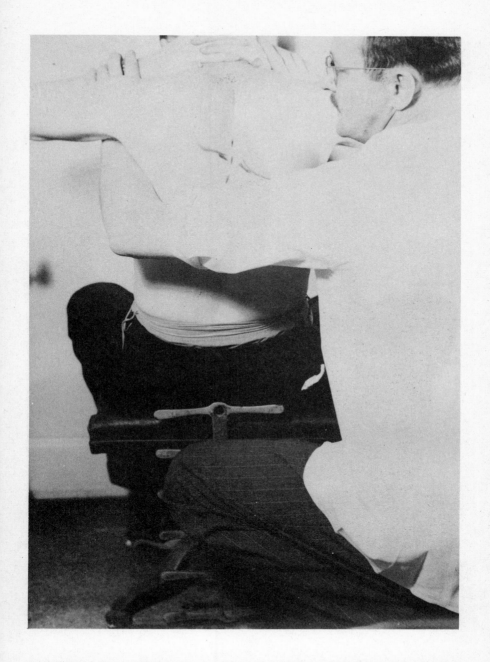

ILLUSTRATING POSITION OF HANDS TO ACQUIRE POSITION-
ING OF PATIENT AND COUNTERFORCE.

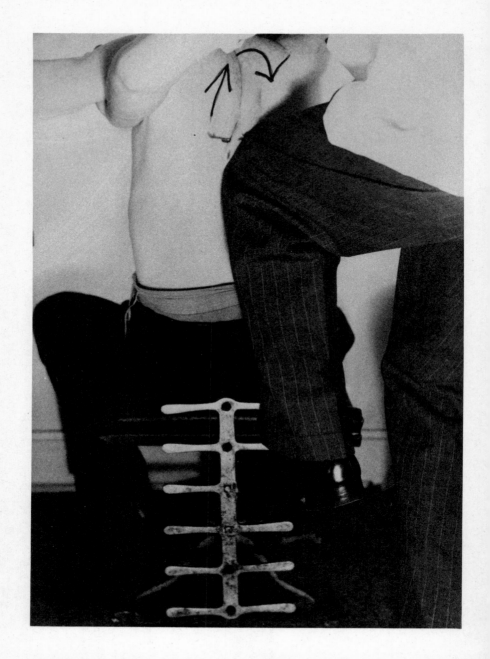

KNEE IS WEDGED BETWEEN APPROXIMATED TRANSVERSE
PROCESSES. PATIENT SLIGHTLY EXTENDED AND LIFTED
FOR COUNTERFORCE.

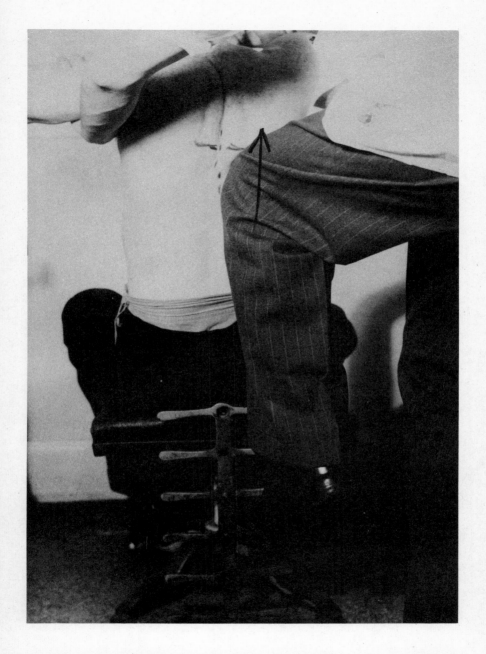

THRUST APPLIED BY RAISING HEEL. THRUST LIFTS SUPER-
IOR SEGMENT ANTERO-SUPERIORLY OFF THE ONE BELOW
UPON WHICH IT WAS EXTENDED.

INSPIRATORY RIB
KNEE TECHNIQUE

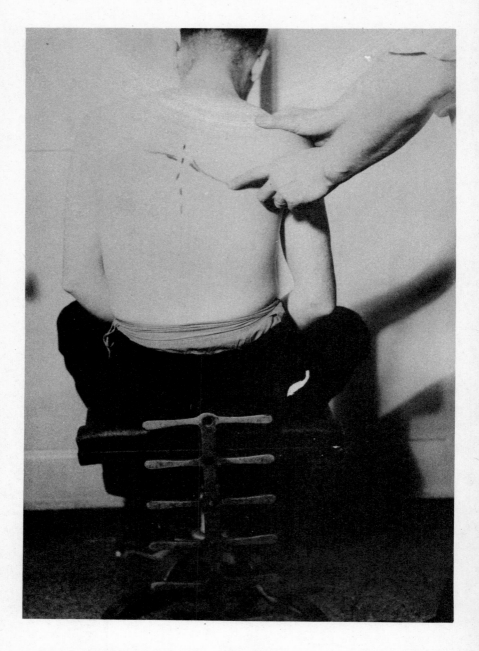

KNEE TECHNIQUE FOR INSPIRATORY RIB. ILLUSTRATING
LOWERED AND PROMINENT ANGLE OF RIB.

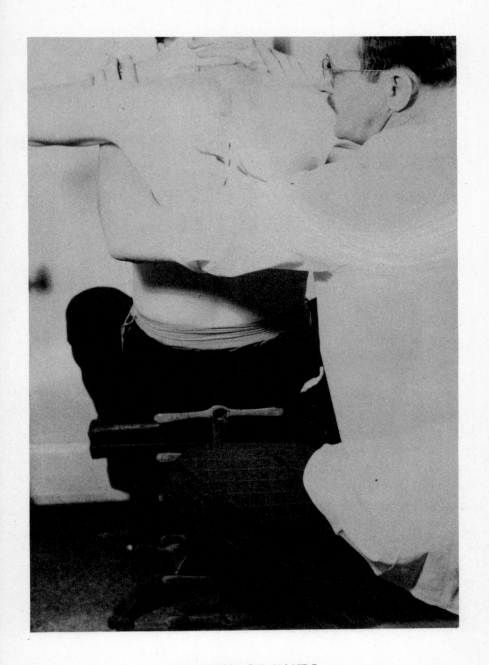

POSITION OF HANDS

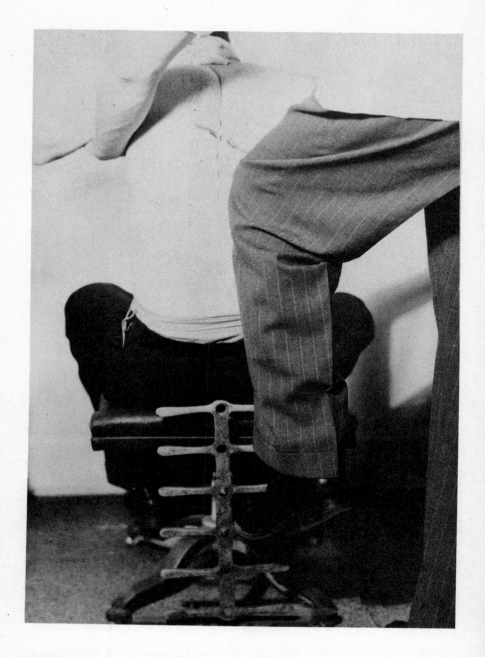

POSITIONING OF PATIENT AND KNEE UNDER THE INSPIR-
ATORY LOWERED RIB ANGLE. PATIENT EXTENDED AND
LIFTED SLIGHTLY FOR COUNTERFORCE.

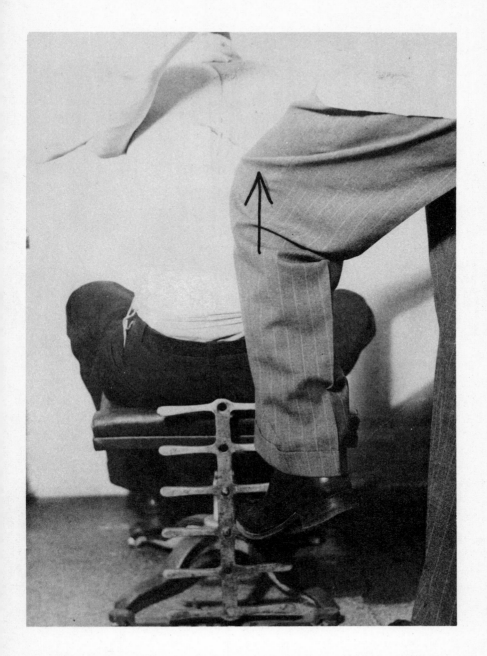

PATIENT FORCIBLY EXHALES WHILE PHYSICIAN THRUSTS RIB ANGLE SUPERIORLY INTO THE EXPIRATORY POSITION TO ESTABLISH FULL MOTION.

CERVICAL AREA

CERVICAL AREA

In the cervical area the plane of the articulations is a continuation upward from the dorsal. The anterosuperiorly directed flattened surfaces are directed toward the chin. They therefore become progressively more horizontal until at the atlanto-axial and occipito-atlantal articulations the plane is parallel with Reids base line, still pointing toward the anatomical position of the chin.

The plane of the articulations requires that corrective forces always approach the chin. In the lower cervical area this necessitates a definite lift in the application of the corrective thrust.

Spinous processes in this area are bifid, irregular, tender, and therefore are poor landmarks to use for diagnostic purposes. Transverse processes similarly are poorly utilized in either diagnosis or treatment.

Articular processes here are fairly symmetrical. They are comparatively superficial; articular processes depict the facet position, the degree of motion present, and serve for the point of contact to administer the corrective force.

Lesions of the cervical segments are charted below up to the atlanto-axial articulation. Lesions of the atlanto-axial and occipito-atlantal area must be considered separately.

Cervical lesions may be favorably influenced by respiratory effort. In inspiration there is a muscular effort on each segment to decrease the anatomically partially extended position. Hence in an extended cervical facet forced inspiration will aid in reducing the degree of extension. Forced expiration will tend to pull the flexed facet into extension position.

Cervical lesions may be found in bilateral flexion, bilateral extension, or more commonly lateral flexion with rotation position.

CERVICAL BILATERAL LESIONS

	BILATERAL EXTENDED FACETS	BILATERAL FLEXED FACETS
Articular processes and facets	Posterior and inferior. Prominent posteriorly.	Antero-superior. Less prominent.
Vertebral body	Tipped postero-inferiorly.	Tipped antero-inferiorly.
Spinous process	Approximates one below. Motion restriction in area of approximation.	Approximates one above. Motion restricted in area of separation.
Vertebra above lesion	Reverse position but mobile. Compensatory.	Compensatory. Reverse position but mobile.

LATERAL FLEXION WITH ROTATION

	EXTENDED FACET SIDE	FLEXED FACET SIDE
Articular process	Posterior-inferior Prominent	Antero-superior Less prominent
Body of vertebra above	Tipped and rotated toward this side.	Tipped and rotated away from this side.
Spinous process	Diverts toward this side.	Diverts toward this side.
Vertebra above lesion	Compensatory. Reversed position but mobile.	Compensatory. Reversed position but mobile.

369

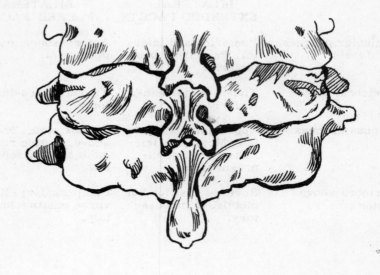

BILATERAL EXTENSION

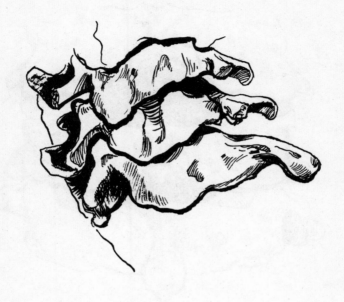

BILATERAL EXTENSION

LATERAL VIEW

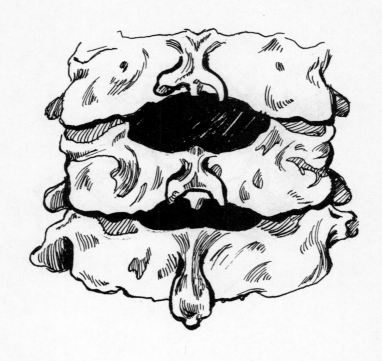

BILATERAL FLEXION

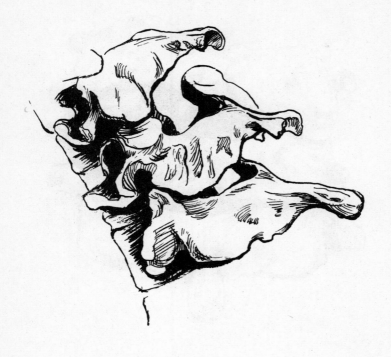

BILATERAL FLEXION

LATERAL VIEW

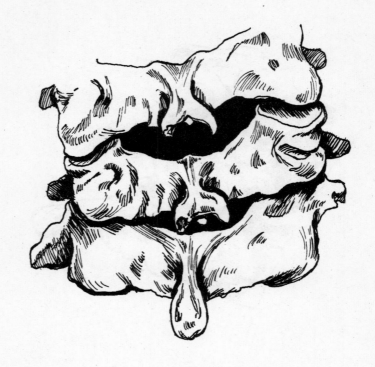

LATERAL FLEXION

WITH ROTATION

CERVICAL TECHNIQUES

EXTENDED FACET
LOWER CERVICAL TECHNIQUE

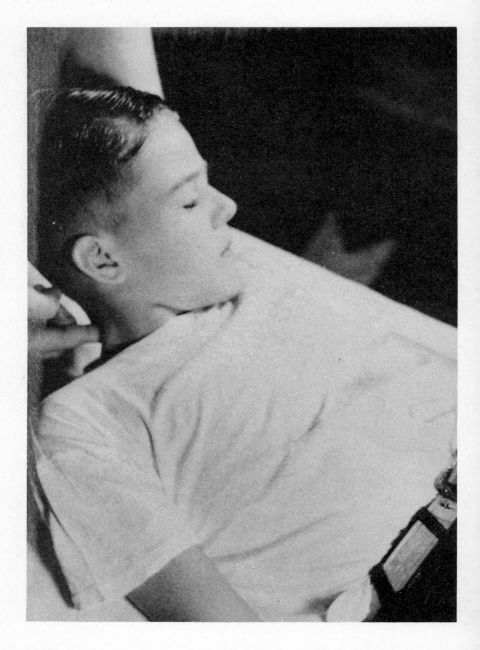

LOWER CERVICAL CORRECTIONS REQUIRE PROGRESSIVELY MORE FLEXION TO LOCK FROM ABOVE DOWN TO THE EX-TENDED ARTICULAR PROCESS.

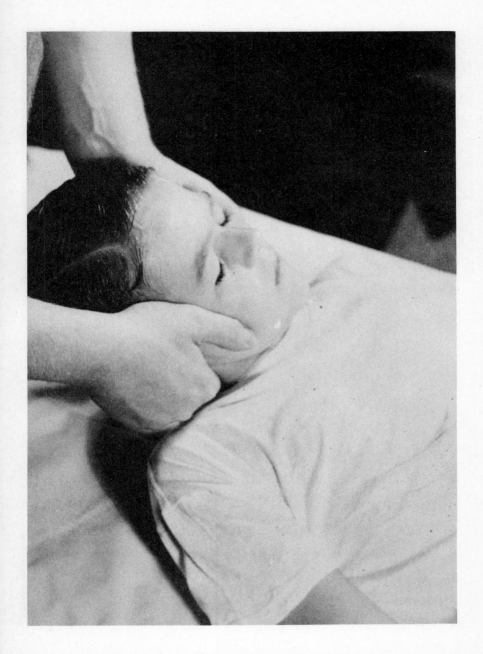

MAINTAINING FLEXION, LATERAL FLEXION ADDED OVER
FINGERS ON EXTENDED PROCESS. ROTATION BY HAND ON
THE ARTICULAR PROCESS CARRIES IT ANTERO-SUPERIORLY
TO THE POINT OF TENSION.

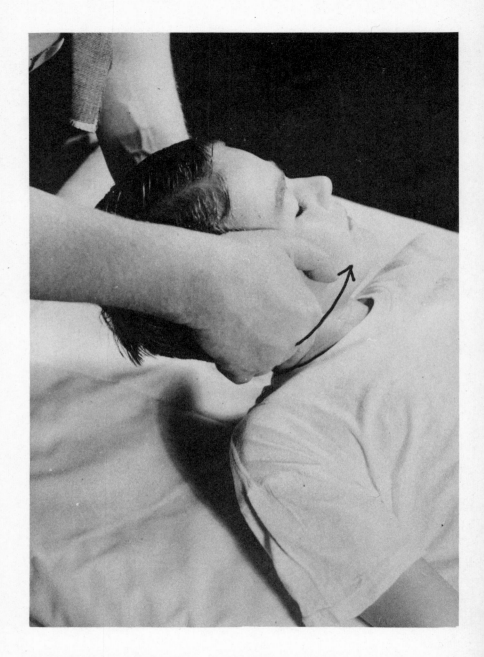

CORRECTIVE THRUST, IF NECESSARY, TOWARD CHIN LIFT-
ING EXTENDED ARTICULAR PROCESS.

EXTENDED FACET
MID CERVICAL TECHNIQUE

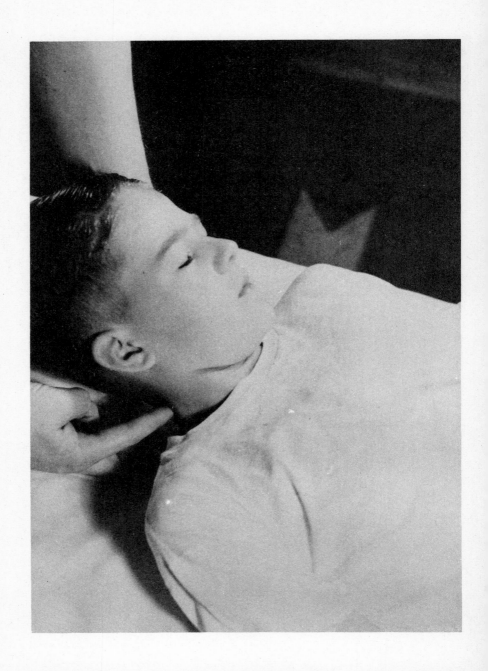

MIDDLE CERVICAL CORRECTIONS REQUIRE SLIGHT FLEXION
DOWN TO EXTENDED ARTICULAR PROCESS.

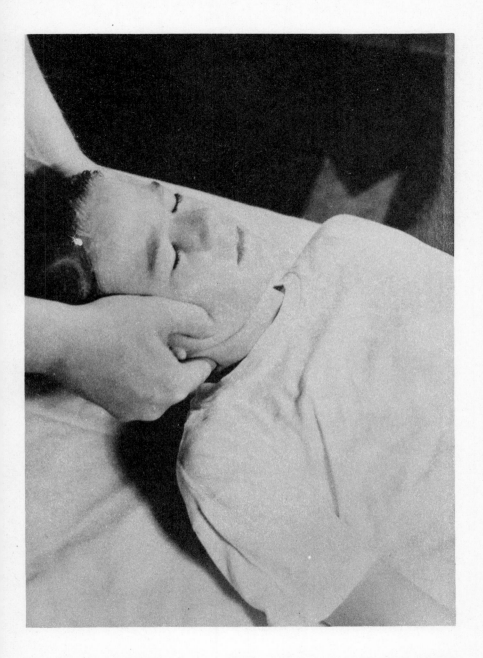

LATERAL FLEXION OVER CORRECTIVE HAND OR FINGERTIPS
FOR COUNTERFORCE.

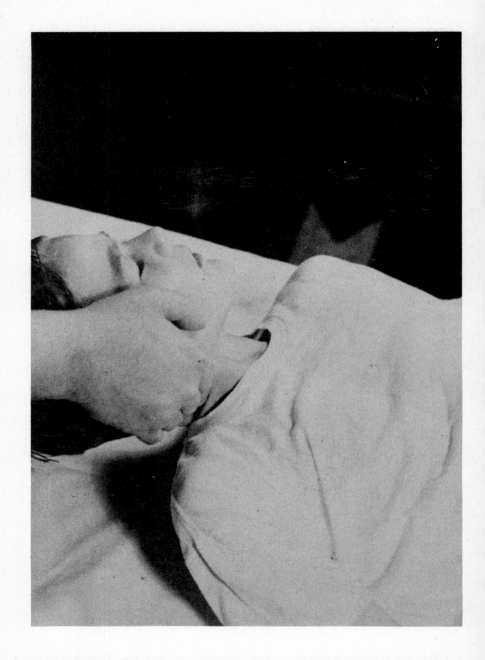

FINGERS ON EXTENDED ARTICULAR PROCESS AND CARRY IT
ANTERO-SUPERIORLY TO NORMAL POSITION. THRUST, IF
ANY, MADE TOWARD CHIN.

ATLANTO - AXIAL AREA

The atlanto-axial articulations are slightly convex, being built up with articular cartilage.

The plane of the articulation is practically horizontal. The motion therefore is almost pure rotation. There is only 5 to 15° of flexion-extension motion. The convex articular surface permit a certain amount of over-riding in rotation. Hence, the atlanto-axial joint has been called a "screw joint". The significance of this anatomical peculiarity is that muscle hypertonicity may impinge those convexities beyond their apex. Without traction to separate the area an attempt to thrust corrective motion may be traumatic. Traction then rotation is the treatment of choice.

Nomenclature suggests the rotated facet, inasmuch as it moves postero-inferior and slightly medially, still be called an extended facet. Lateral flexion with rotation will then apply in the atlanto-axial area.

LATERAL FLEXION WITH ROTATION

	EXTENDED FACET SIDE	FLEXED FACET SIDE
Upper segment with relation to lower body of vertebra	Rotates toward this side	Rotates from this side
Spinous tubercle	Shifts to opposite side	Shifts toward this side
Articular Process	Posterior and prominent	Anterior and less prominent
Transverse process	Posterior	Anterior

ATLANTO AXIAL
EXTENDED FACET TECHNIQUE

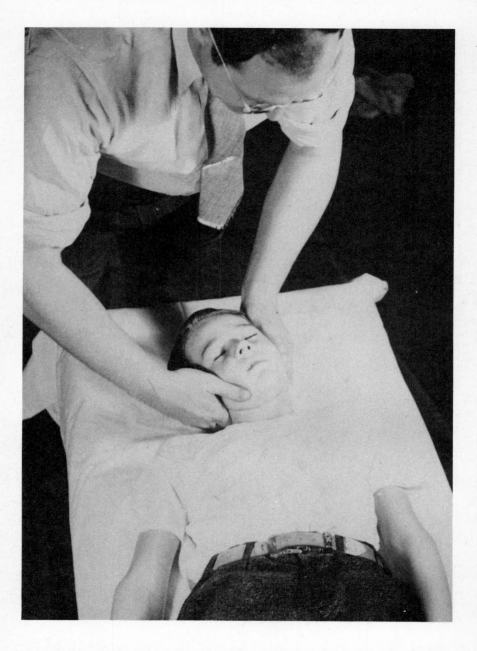

EXTENDED ATLAS ARCH FIXED WITH CORRECTIVE HAND.
LATERAL FLEXION FOR COUNTERFORCE.

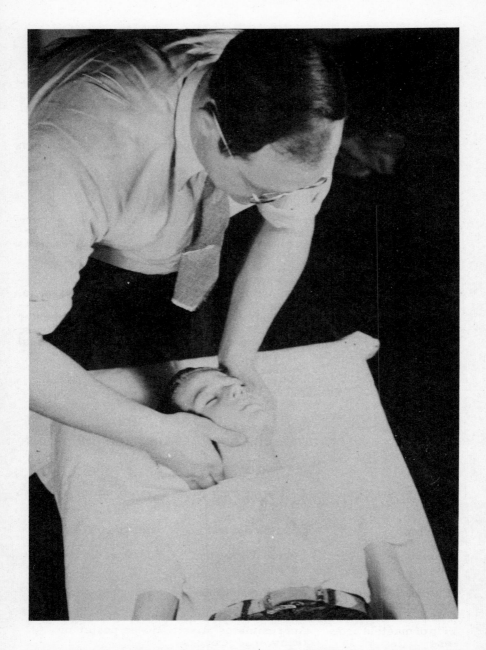

HAND CARRIES EXTENDED ATLAS ANTERIORLY ON AXIS BY
ALMOST PURE ROTATION.

OCCIPITO-ATLANTAL AREA

This articulation is made by the knob like condyle of the occiput, that is received into the concave postero-laterally diverging and laterally raised margin of the articular surface on the lateral mass of the atlas.

All motions are free in flexion, extension, or lateral flexion with rotation.

The articular plane is horizontal, hence corrective forces should be toward the chin.

Occipito-atlantal lesions are found restrained by the physiological positions of bilateral flexion, bilateral extension, or lateral flexion with rotation. Chart of the diagnostic positional relations will be found below.

A word of caution seems necessary inasmuch as the occipito-atlantal lesions are the most frequently found in the spinal area. They are also the most prone to recur. Probably 95% of all occipito-atlantal lesions are maintained by reflex arc disturbances or compensatory mechanics, and frequently both. Treatment of these factors is as essential as is the correction of the occipito-atlantal lesion responsible for them or resulting from them.

OCCIPITO-ATLANTAL LESIONS

	BILATERAL EX-TENDED CONDYLES	BILATERALLY FLEXED CONDYLES
Condyles	Move anterior	Move Posterior
Atlas arch	Left prominent posteriorly	Less prominent
Occiput	Slips forward	Slips posterior
Basilar process	Forward and upward	Postero-inferior
External Occipital protruberance	Anterior and inferior	Postero-superior
Tip of mastoid process	Approximates atlas transverse process	Moves posterior
Angle of mandible	Moves anterior from transverse process	Approximates transverse process
Chin	Elevates	Depresses

LATERAL FLEXION WITH ROTATION LESIONS

	EXTENDED CONDYLAR SIDE	FLEXED CONDYLAR SIDE
Condyle	Anterior	Posterior
Atlas Arch	Prominent	Less prominent
Occiput	Slips from and tilts toward this side	Slips toward and tilts away from flexed condylar side.
Top of head	Tips toward this side	Tips away from this side
Chin	Rotates from extended condylar side	Rotates toward flexed condylar side.
Tip of mastoid	Approximates transverse process	Moves posterior from transverse process
Angle of mandible	Moves anteriorly from transverse process	Approximates transverse process.
Transverse process of Atlas	Prominent	Less prominent

OCCIPITO-ATLANTAL
EXTENDED CONDYLAR TECHNIQUE

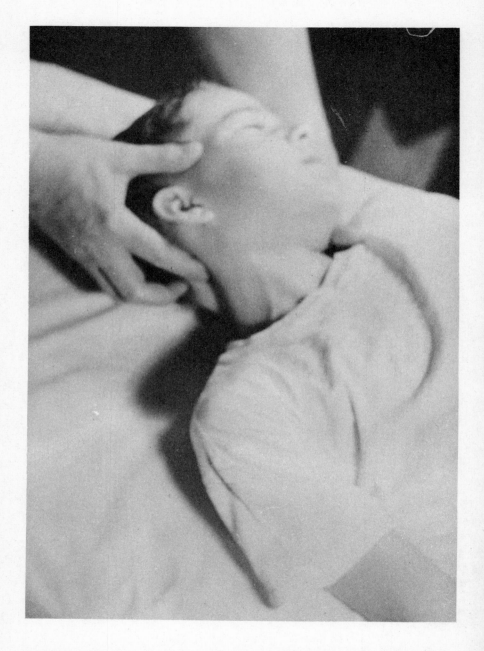

FINGER ON ATLAS ARCH ON SIDE OF EXTENDED CONDYLE.

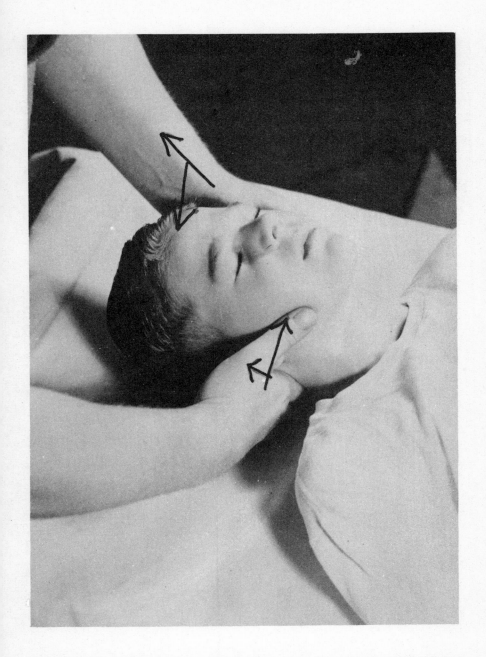

CORRECTIVE HAND PLACED ON ATLAS ARCH, LATERAL
FLEXION FOR COUNTERFORCE.

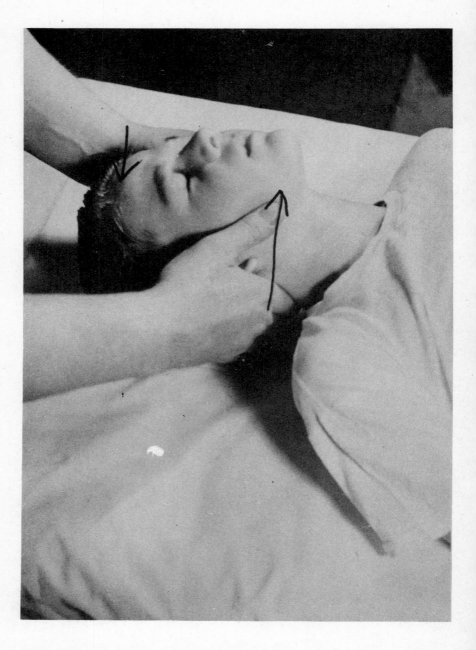

CORRECTIVE HAND CARRIES ATLAS ARCH ANTERIORLY UN-
DER OCCIPUT. THRUST IS TOWARD THE CHIN.

FLEXED CONDYLAR SIDE
TYPICAL CERVICAL TECHNIQUE

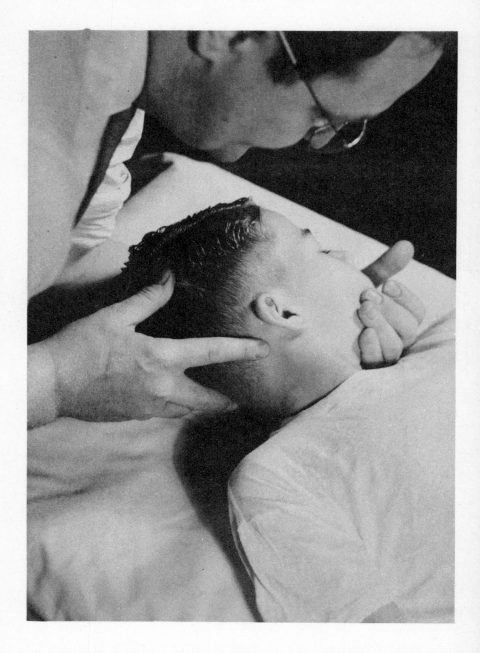

PALPATING POSTERO-LATERALLY RESTRICTED FLEXED
CONDYLAR AREA.

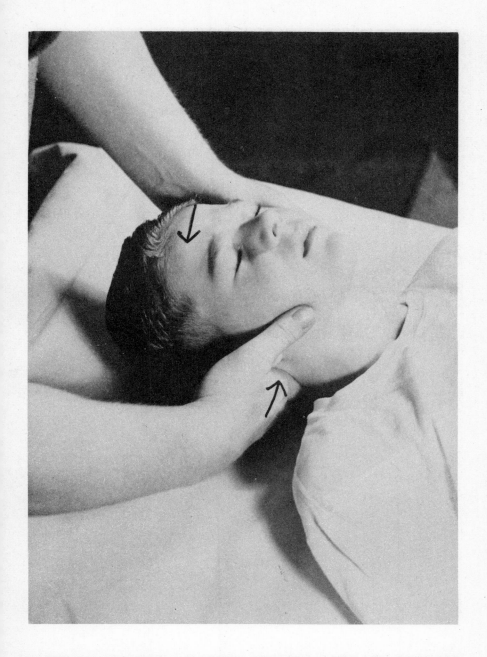

LATERAL FLEXION OF HEAD AGAINST HAND ON MASTOID
PROCESS.

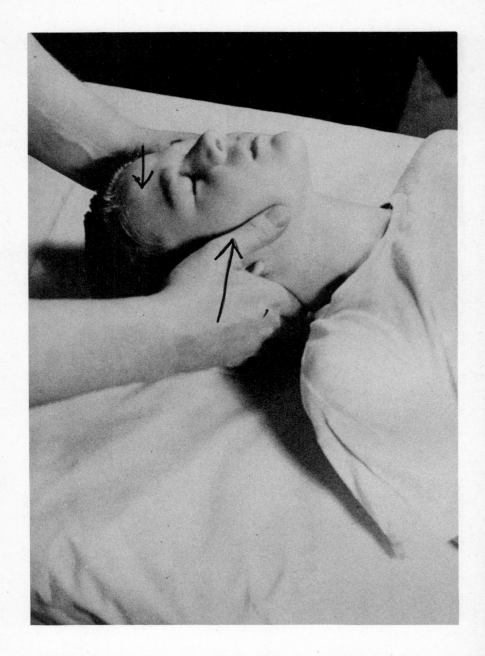

CORRECTIVE ROTATION ON MASTOID CARRYING FLEXED
CONDYLAR SIDE ANTERIOR TOWARD EXTENDED POSITION.

OCCIPITO ATLANTAL
FLEXED CONDYLAR TECHNIQUE

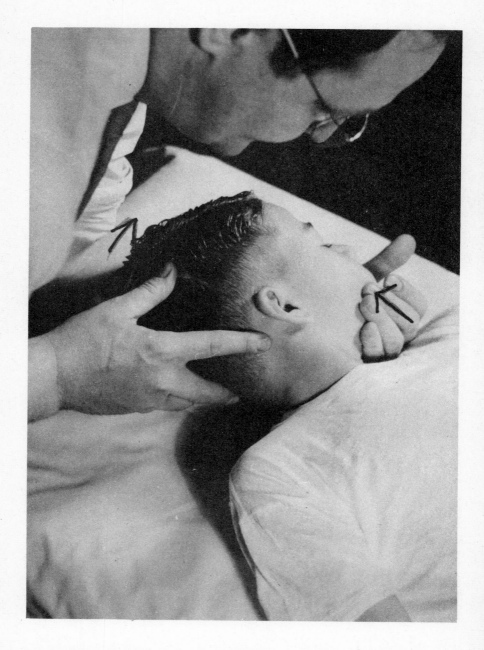

HEAD SUPPORTED ON ARM, HAND CUPPING CHIN FOR TRAC-
TION.

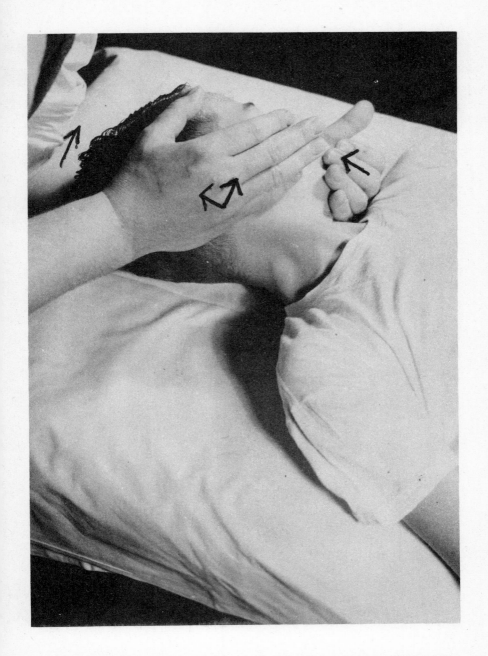

HYPOTHENAR EMINENCE PLACED ON MASTOID PROCESS.

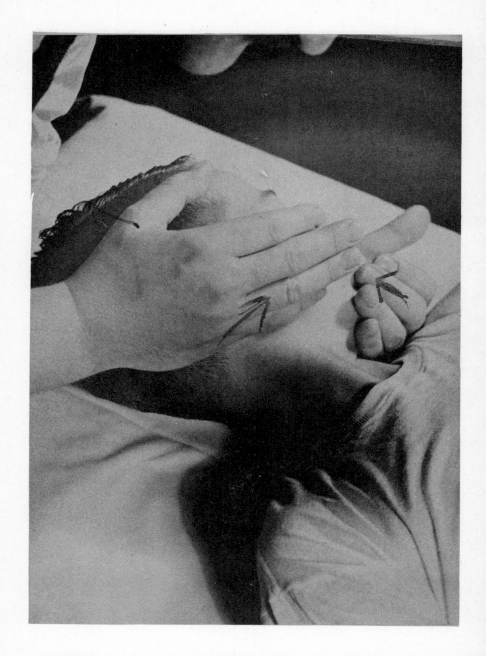

TRACTION, LATERAL FLEXION, AND ROTATION INSTITUTED
TO MOVE FLEXED CONDYLE ANTERIORLY. THRUST IS MADE
IN TRACTION AND ANTERIORLY ON MASTOID PROCESS.

SHOULDER GIRDLE

AND

UPPER EXTREMITY

SHOULDER GIRDLE

Most lesions of the shoulder area are usually found to be of the acromio-clavicular articulation, deltoid bursa or muscle, supraspinatus muscle, 1st rib, cervical anomaly, anterior scalenus, or neuritis instead of the true shoulder articulation itself. The shoulder joint itself is similar to the true hip joint. The great range of motion renders simple synovitis a very infrequent involvement. Whenever pain and/or muscle spasm impair joint motion one should always anticipate serious joint disease.

The shallow glenoid labrum, great amount of shoulder girdle musculature and the interposed clavicle, all however make the shoulder area susceptible to strain and trauma.

After ruling out true shoulder joint disease one must direct treatment to the shoulder area in general and also to the specific etiological factor, usually one of these listed above but may be other less frequent found factors. In this manual we are concerned only with the manipulative phase of the management of the above conditions.

Palpation of the shoulder areas will reveal muscle hypertonicities, atrophies, malpositions due to compensatory mechanics and also those due to reflex and traumatic factors.

Muscle relaxation of the shoulder girdle must be thorough and mild. Motion is carried only to the point of pain. Cervico-dorsal area is reflexly and mechanically related.

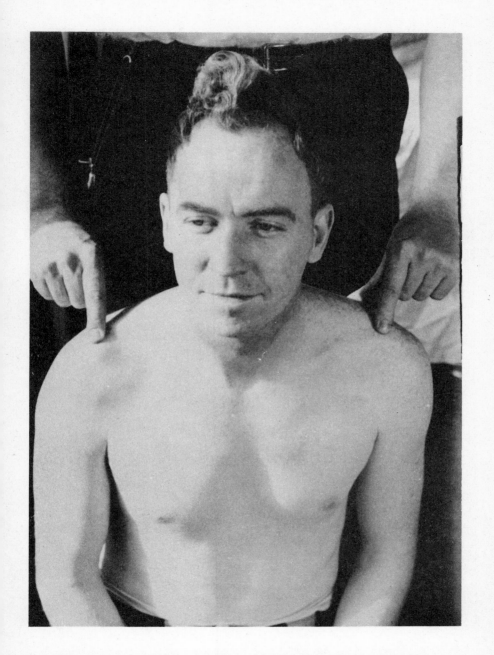

PALPATING COMPARATIVE PROMINENCE OF ACROMIUM, CLAVICLE, AND JOINT SPACE.

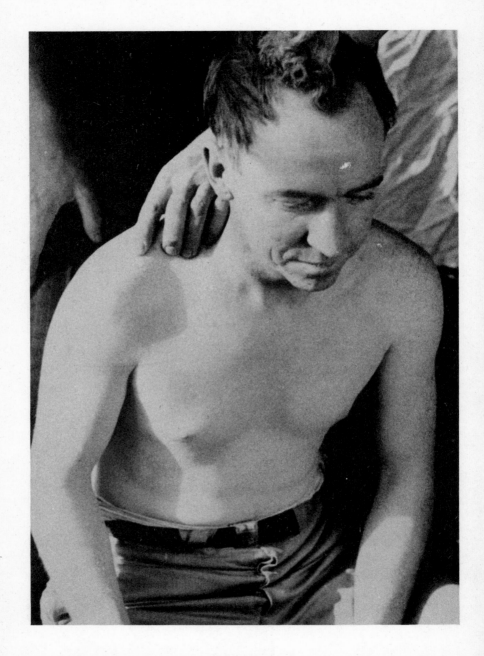

LESION LOCATED, WITH PAIN, SWELLING, TRAJECTORY PAR-
ESTHESIAS, FIBROSIS ETC.

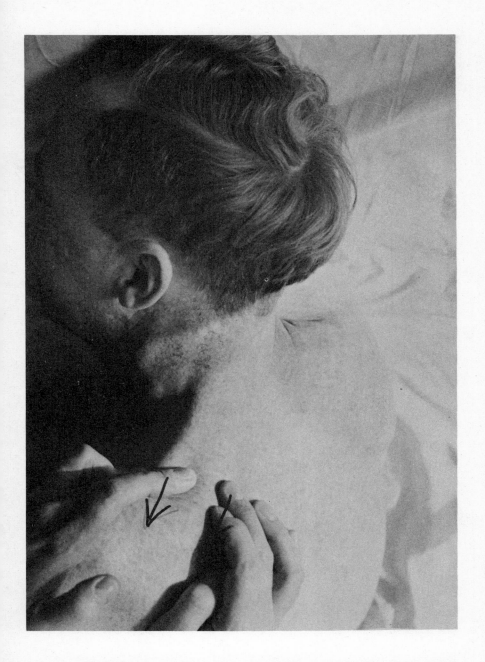

GENERAL SHOULDER GIRDLE RELAXATION SHOULD PRECEDE
SPECIFIC LESION CORRECTION. LEVATOR ANGULAE SCAPU-
LAE, TRAPEZIUS, AND SUPRA-SPINATUS MUSCLES STRETCHED
AND RELAXED.

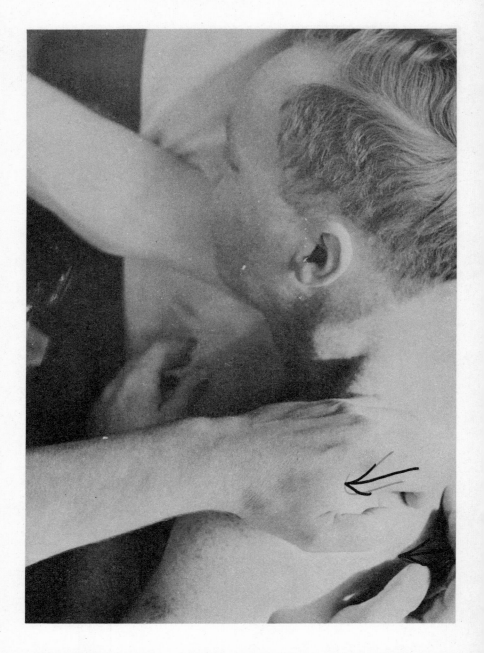

RHOMBOIDEI STRETCHED BY PULLING SCAPULA LATERALLY.

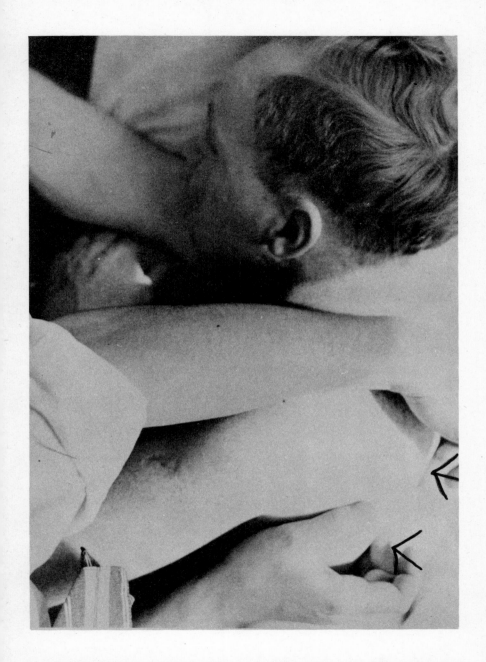

RHOMBOIDEI AND SUBSCAPULARIS TREATED BY SEPARATING
SCAPULA FROM POSTERIOR THORACIC WALL.

ACROMIO-CLAVICULAR LESIONS

CLAVICULAR ASCENT

Clavicular ascent or "dropped shoulder" is usually due to a trauma that carries the acromion process inferiorly and under the articulating surface of the clavicle. Clavicle then remains more prominent than the acromion process and its fellow on the opposite side.

Shoulder area is frequently carried "en masse" high to facilitate return circulation and comfort even tho the acromion and scapula are "dropped" with relation to the clavicle.

Treatment should include muscle relaxation, separation of the articulation, and corrective force to depress the distal clavicle.

Application of tape to take the pull off the brachial plexus and the deltoid muscle usually is valuable. Cervico-dorsal area must be managed also.

CLAVICULAR ASCENT
TECHNIQUE FOR CORRECTION

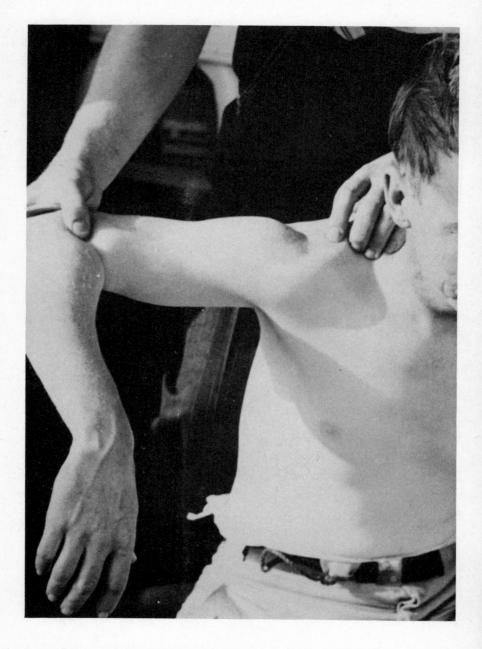

CLAVICULAR ASCENT- ARM RAISED TO PERMIT KNEE OR PILLOW TO BE INSERTED INTO AXILLARY SPACE.

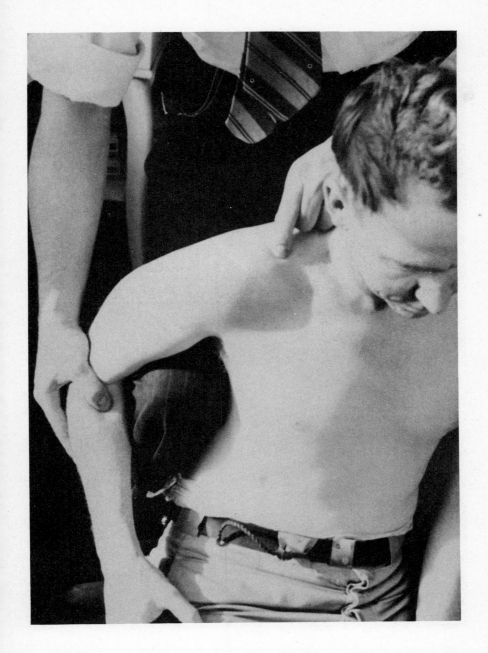

KNEE OR PILLOW IN AXILLARY SPACE, ARM IS ADDUCTED
OVER SUCH PROMINENCE TO GAP THE ACROMIO-CLAVICULAR
JOINT.

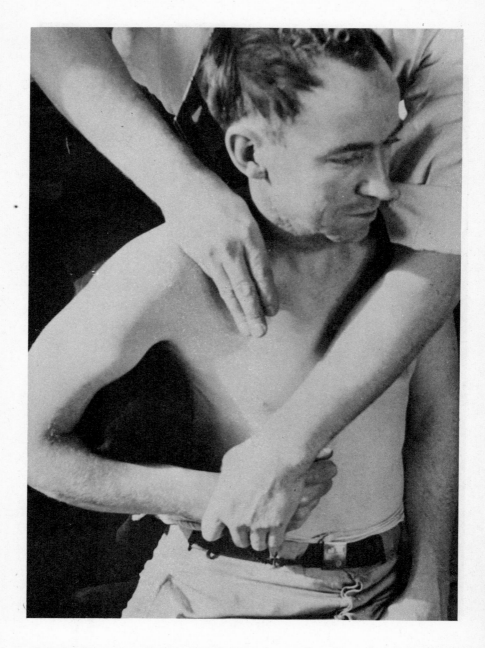

WITH JOINT GAPPED-DISTAL END OF CLAVICLE IS FORCED
ANTERO-INFERIORLY TO NORMAL POSITION.

CLAVICULAR DESCENT

Clavicular descent is just the reverse of clavicular ascent and requires force in the opposite direction for correction.

Clavicular descent may be acquired by a downward force on the distal clavicle or an upward jerk on the arm that will elevate the acromion process.

Palpation compares the decreased motion, pain etc. in the involved articular area with the normal fellow. The distal clavicle is lessened in superior prominence and the acromium is more superficial.

Treatment consists of gapping the articulations and rolling the humerus and scapula while the other hand elevates the distal end of the clavicle.

Cervico-dorsal area must be managed also.

CLAVICULAR DESCENT

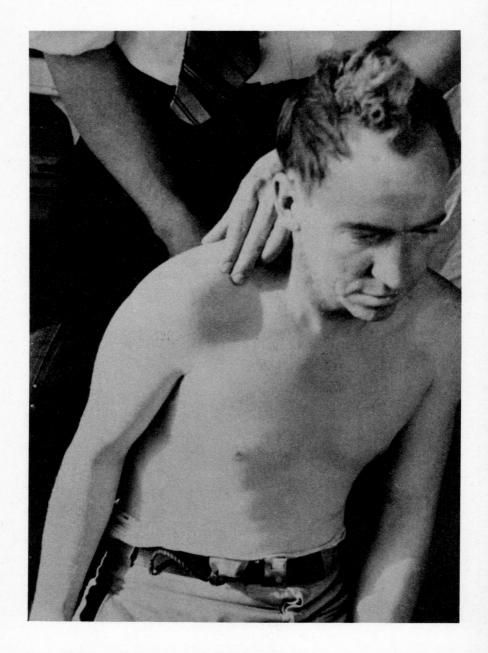

PALPATING PROMINENT ACROMIUM, AND DECREASED CLAV-
ICULAR PROMINENCE IN CLAVICULAR DESCENT.

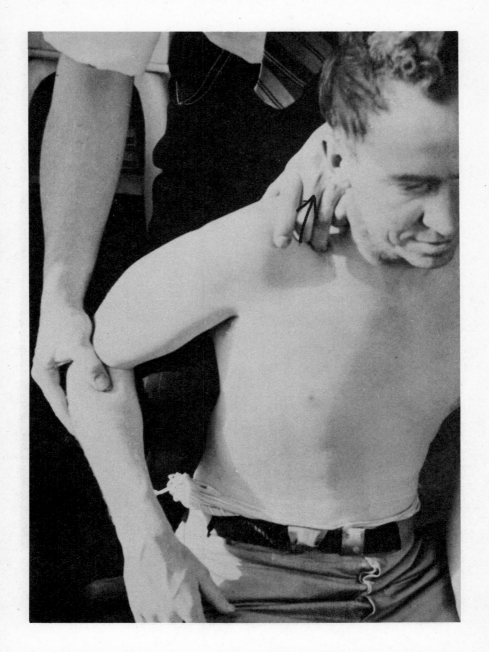

FINGER PADS INSERTED UNDER DISTAL END OF CLAVICLE
TO ELEVATE IT TO NORMAL POSITION. OTHER HAND BE-
GINS ROTATION AND CIRCUMDUCTION OF ARM TO OPEN
ACROMIO-CLAVICULAR ARTICULATION.

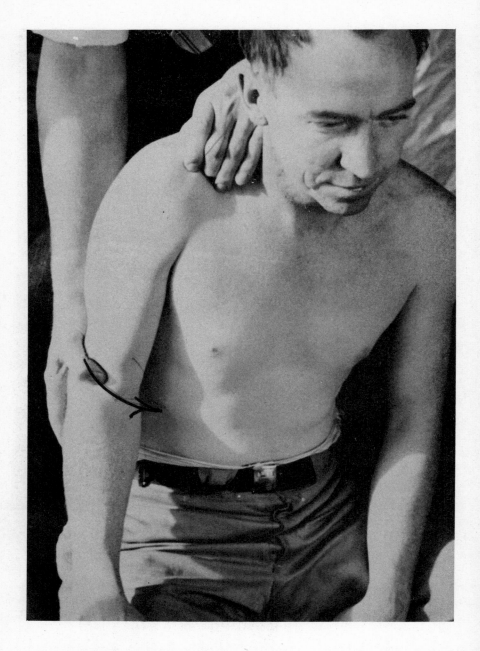

ARM STARTED ACROSS MIDLINE TO GAP ARTICULATION BY
COMPLETE ADDUCTION.

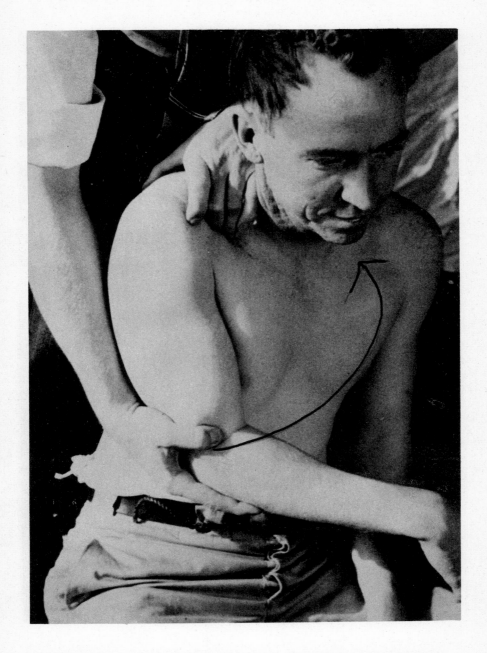

ADDUCTION COMPLETE, LIFT ON CLAVICLE MAINTAINED.

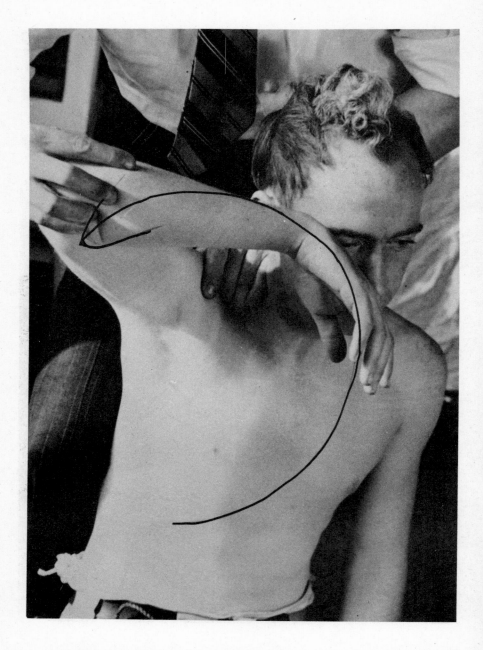

CIRCUMDUCTION-COMPLETE LIFT ON CLAVICLE MAIN-
TAINED.

RADIO-ULNAR HUMERAL LESION

(TENNIS ELBOW)

Usually an external rotation is responsible for traumatizing all these articulations. In addition, the pronator muscle tissue is inflamed primarily or secondarily. Hence the patient finds pain or difficulty in extending the forearm or in externally rotating the forearm or both.

External rotation angulates the ulna with the proximal end slipping medially and the distal end laterally.

The hypertonic pronator maintains a posterior positioning of the proximal radius and an anterior mal-alignment of the distal radial end.

Local treatment should relax the musculature and reverse the position of the mal-alignment. Cervico-dorsal area is usually reflexly related.

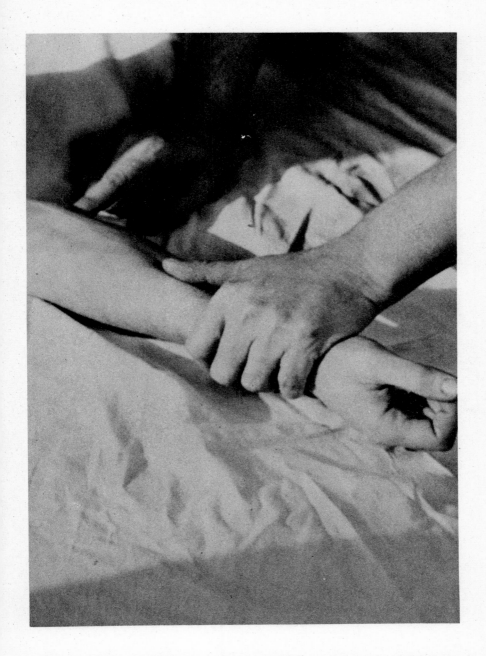

RADIO-ULNAR HUMERAL LESION (TENNIS ELBOW) PROXIMAL
END OF ULNA PALPATED, ARM EXTENDED. DISTAL END OF
FORE-ARM HELD BY OTHER HAND.

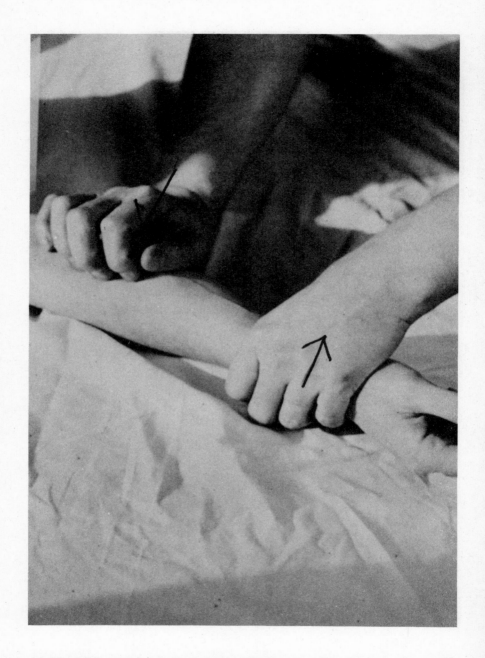

HEEL OF HAND APPLIED TO PROXIMAL END OF ULNA. ARM,
AND FOREARM FLAT ON TABLE, ROTATION OF RADIUS 45°.

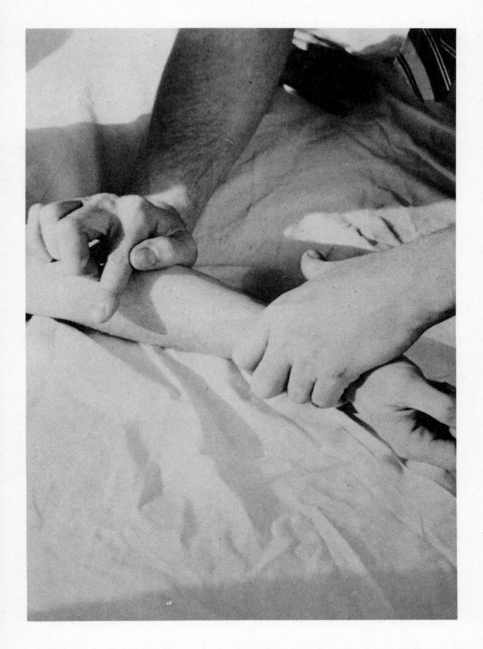

LATERAL THRUST MADE ON PROXIMAL RADIUS. COUNTER-
FORCE BY OPPOSITE HAND ON PATIENT'S FORE-ARM DIS-
TALLY.

POSTERIOR PROXIMAL RADIUS
RADIO-ULNAR LESION

The radius at its proximal end is posterior and prominent. Pain is usually marked on use and when the area is accidently brushed against a hard object.

Supporting the proximal radius posteriorly, then hyperextending the forearm with slight force and great care will usually reposition the malalignment. Local treatment for the muscle tissue and the cervico-dorsal area is also indicated.

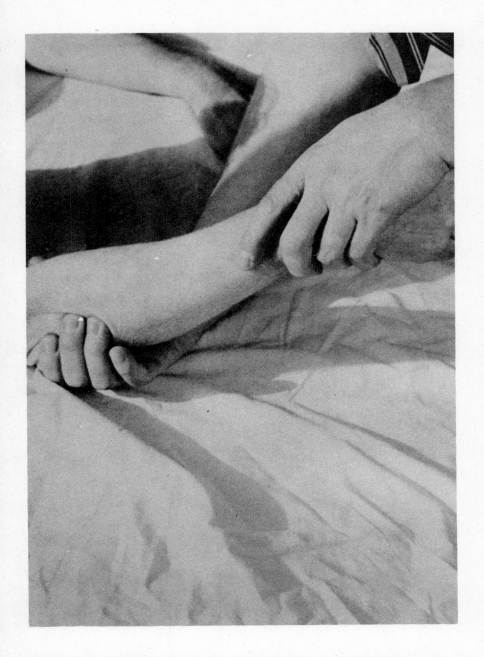

POSTERIOR RADIAL HEAD - POSTERIOR AND PROMINENT RA-
DIAL HEAD IS LOCATED. SEVERAL FINGERS ARE PLACED
ON A LINE DISTAL TO IT.

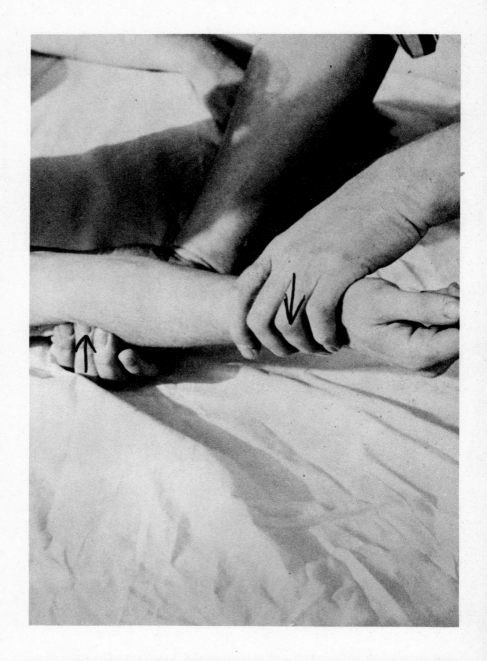

HAND ON WRIST PREVENTS PRONATION OF HAND AND BEGINS
HYPEREXTENSION OF ELBOW.

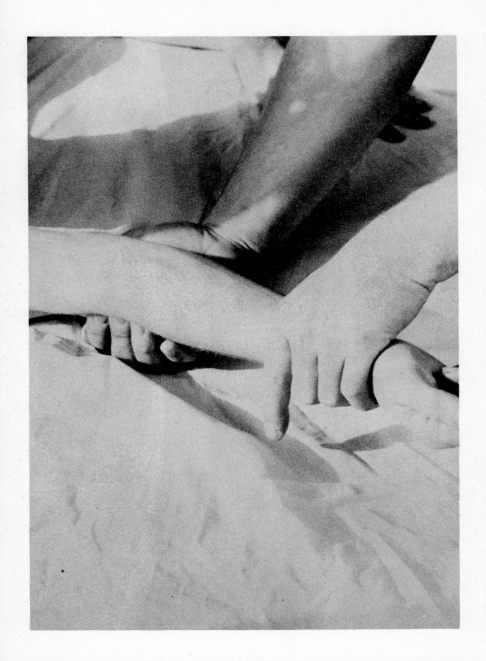

MILD BUT QUICK HYPER-EXTENSION OVER THE FINGERS
FORCES THE RADIAL HEAD ANTERIORLY TO NORMAL POSI-
TION. PASSIVE MOTION SHOULD BE EXERCISED FREELY.